T0226678

Cytopathology

Editor

TARIK M. ELSHEIKH

SURGICAL PATHOLOGY CLINICS

surgpath.theclinics.com

Consulting Editor
JOHN R. GOLDBLUM

March 2014 • Volume 7 • Number 1

ELSEVIER

1600 John F. Kennedy Boulevard • Suite 1800 • Philadelphia, Pennsylvania, 19103-2899

http://www.theclinics.com

SURGICAL PATHOLOGY CLINICS Volume 7, Number 1
March 2014 ISSN 1875-9181, ISBN-13: 978-0-323-26132-6

Editor: Joanne Husovski
Developmental Editor: Donald Mumford

Surgical Pathology Clinics (ISSN 1875-9181) is published quarterly by Elsevier Inc., 360 Park Avenue South, New York, NY 10010. Months of issue are March, June, September, and December. Business and Editorial Office: Elsevier Inc., 1600 John F. Kennedy Blvd., Ste. 1800, Philadelphia, PA 19103-2899. Accounting and Circulation Offices: Elsevier Inc., 3251 Riverport Lane, Maryland Heights, MO 63043. Periodicals postage paid at New York, NY and at additional mailing offices. Subscription prices are $200.00 per year (US individuals), $233.00 per year (US institutions), $100.00 per year (US students/residents), $250.00 per year (Canadian individuals), $266.00 per year (Canadian Institutions), $250.00 per year (foreign individuals), $266.00 per year (foreign institutions), and $120.00 per year (international & Canadian students/residents). Foreign air speed delivery is included in all *Clinics'* subscription prices. All prices are subject to change without notice. **POSTMASTER:** Send address changes to *Surgical Pathology Clinics*, Elsevier, 3251 Riverport Lane, Maryland Heights, MO 63043. Customer Service: 1-800-654-2452 (US). From outside the United States, call 1-314-447-8871. Fax: 1-314-447-8029. E-mail: JournalsCustomerServiceusa@elsevier.com (for print support) and JournalsOnlineSupport-usa@elsevier.com (for online support).

Reprints. For copies of 100 or more, of articles in this publication, please contact the Commercial Reprints Department, Elsevier Inc., 360 Park Avenue South, New York, NY 10010-1710. Tel. 212-633-3874; Fax: 212-633-3820; E-mail: reprints@elsevier.com.

Contributors

CONSULTING EDITOR

JOHN R. GOLDBLUM, MD
Chairman, Professor of Pathology, Department
of Anatomic Pathology, Cleveland Clinics
Lerner College of Medicine, Cleveland Clinic,
Cleveland, Ohio

EDITOR

TARIK M. ELSHEIKH, MD
Medical Director of Anatomic Pathology
Services Cleveland Clinic Laboratories
Cleveland, Ohio

AUTHORS

KRISTEN ATKINS, MD
Associate Professor, Department of
Pathology, University of Virginia,
Charlottesville, Virginia

BARBARA A. CENTENO, MD
Director of Cytology and Anatomic Pathology
Quality Assurance, H. Lee Moffitt Cancer
Center and Research Institute, Professor of
Oncologic Sciences and Pathology and Cell
Biology, Morsani College of Medicine,
University of South Florida, Tampa, Florida

EDIZ F. COSAR, MD
Department of Pathology, University of
Massachusetts Medical School, Worcester,
Massachusetts

DAVID J. DABBS, MD
Professor, Chief of Pathology at Magee
Women's Hospital, Department of Pathology,
University of Pittsburgh Medical Center,
Pittsburgh, Pennsylvania

LLOYD M. HUTCHINSON, PhD
Department of Pathology, University of
Massachusetts Medical School, Worcester,
Massachusetts

SUSANNE JEFFUS, MD
Assistant Professor, Department of
Pathology, University of Arkansas, Little Rock,
Arkansas

JOSÉ CARLOS MACHADO, PhD
Associate Professor of Pathology at Medical
Faculty of Porto University; Senior Researcher
IPATIMUP, Institute of Molecular Pathology
and Immunology of Porto University, Porto,
Portugal

SARA E. MONACO, MD
Associate Professor, Director of FNA Service at
Children's Hospital of Pittsburgh, Program
Director of UPMC Cytopathology Fellowship,
Department of Pathology, University of
Pittsburgh Medical Center, Pittsburgh,
Pennsylvania

N. PAUL OHORI, MD
Professor of Pathology, Medical Director of
Cytopathology, Department of Pathology,
University of Pittsburgh Medical Center -
Presbyterian, Pittsburgh, Pennsylvania

MICHELLE D. REID, MD, MS
Associate Professor of Pathology, Emory
University, Atlanta, Georgia

FERNANDO SCHMITT, MD, PhD, FIAC
Professor of Pathology, Department of
Laboratory Medicine and Pathobiology, Faculty
of Medicine, University of Toronto, Toronto,
Ontario, Canada; Senior Researcher IPATIMUP,
Institute of Molecular Pathology and
Immunology of Porto University, Porto, Portugal

KAREN E. SCHOEDEL, MD
Associate Professor of Pathology, University of
Pittsburgh Medical Center - Presbyterian,
Pittsburgh, Pennsylvania

RAJA R. SEETHALA, MD
Department of Pathology, University of
Pittsburgh Medical Center, Pittsburgh,
Pennsylvania

AMY G. ZHOU, MD
Department of Pathology, University of
Massachusetts Medical School, Worcester,
Massachusetts

Contents

Fine-needle aspiration biopsy of the pancreas is indicated for sampling of solid and cystic masses. Preoperative cytologic diagnosis of pancreatic ductal adenocarcinoma and cystic lesions on cytology can be problematic, and ancillary studies may help confirm diagnosis. Ancillary studies in pancreatic cytology include special stains, immunohistochemistry, mutational analyses of specific genes, cyst fluid analysis of tumor markers and enzymes, and, in some instances, flow cytometry. Proteomics, microRNA sequencing, and whole-exome gene sequencing have been used to illustrate the progression of pancreatic neoplasms and identify key diagnostic markers. This article summarizes recent literature on ancillary studies in pancreatic fine-needle aspiration samples.

The importance of cytologic techniques for investigation of respiratory conditions has been recognized since the earliest days of clinical cytology. Cytology is able to detect most of mycoses and parasitic and viral infections based on the morphologic recognition of these agents. The most relevant application of lung cytology today is in the diagnosis and management of lung cancer; approximately 70% of those cancers are diagnosed at a late stage and are unresectable. This article addresses the most common ancillary techniques, such as special stains, immunocytochemistry, and molecular testing, used to refine the cytologic diagnosis of lung cancer and to guide personalized therapy.

Recent advances in thyroid imaging, clinical evaluation, cytopathology, surgical pathology, and molecular diagnostics have contributed toward greater understanding of thyroid nodules. In particular, the development of the Bethesda System for Reporting Thyroid Cytopathology (BSRTC) has brought standardization to the field and the system dovetails well with the implementation of immunohistochemistry and molecular testing to diagnostic practice. Among the molecular strategies available, the application of the molecular panel of common genetic alterations can stratify indeterminate BSRTC diagnoses into low-risk and high-risk groups. The molecular panel markers have a high positive predictive value and therefore, the panel is considered to be a "rule-in" test. In contrast, the Afirma gene expression classifier by Veracyte Corporation is a test that has been reported to have a high negative predictive value, and therefore, considered to be a "rule-out" test. With further advances, refinements are expected to be made. In particular, the application of next-generation sequencing technology holds promise in bringing thyroid cytopathology to the next level.

Common usage of fine-needle aspirate (FNA) for salivary gland lesions is the preoperative determination of whether a lesion is neoplastic, its lineage, and if neoplastic, whether it is low grade/benign, or high grade. Immunohistochemical stains can be performed on cell blocks to determine lineage and help refine diagnosis, although their performance is not always equivalent to that seen in surgical specimens. Several characteristic translocations have been described in various entities in these categories, and these can be evaluated using fluorescence in situ hybridization. In the future, high-throughput next-generation sequencing panels may further refine cytologic diagnosis in salivary tumors.

Urothelial carcinoma (UC) is the most common malignancy of the urinary tract. Cytology and cystoscopy are two of the most commonly used tests for screening and diagnosis of UC. However, the sensitivity of cytology for UC is less than ideal, while cystoscopy is an invasive and expensive procedure. The search for an accurate, sensitive, noninvasive, and cost-effective method for detecting UC has led to the development of ancillary studies using immunological and molecular methods.

Cytology has been the mainstay of cervical dysplasia and cancer screening in the United States. The specificity of a woman harboring a high-grade lesion when identified as high-grade squamous intraepithelial lesion on Pap test is high; however, the test suffers from low sensitivity. Epidemiology studies have demonstrated that human papillomavirus (HPV) types 16 and 18 account for most cervical squamous cell carcinomas. Tests have been developed to identify high-risk HPV, some specifically to identify HPV 16 and 18. Simultaneous to the increase in HPV detection methods, interdisciplinary groups are making recommendations on the managerial use of the tests.

The application of ancillary studies, such as immunostains, to cytopathology has improved the ability to make accurate diagnoses with precise subclassification. Even with these techniques, there are still aspiration and exfoliative cytology cases for which it remains difficult to definitively determine the source and/or subtype. This article focuses on the well-established and novel ancillary studies used in the modern era of cancer diagnoses in cytopathology, particularly in the diagnostic work-up of metastatic tumors without a known primary.

SURGICAL PATHOLOGY CLINICS

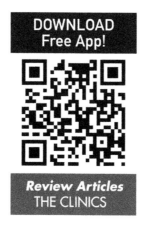

Preface
Cytology: Moving Forward!

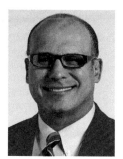

Tarik M. Elsheikh, MD
Editor

The utility of ancillary studies, such as special stains, immunohistochemistry, and molecular testing in the workup of malignant and premalignant disease, has added a new dimension to the field of pathology. As pathologists, we are continuously asked today to make more specific diagnoses from smaller samples. In this capacity, cytology has evolved to play an integral role in the diagnosis and management of oncologic diseases. No longer is a cytologic diagnosis just about reporting the presence or absence of malignant cells; rather it is now about making a precise and definitive diagnosis. Clinicians increasingly request information regarding specific classification of the malignant tumors, and in many cases, application of additional prognostic and therapeutic markers to help guide their clinical management. Although morphology remains the cornerstone of cytology, ancillary studies can confirm and/or subclassify a malignancy in many cases. In some instances a malignant or premalignant diagnosis can only be rendered after incorporating the findings of both cytomorphology and ancillary studies.

Although most pathologists recognize the critical role of ancillary testing, it can be extremely frustrating for many of us to keep up with the new advances and rapidly growing developments in the fields of immunohistochemistry and molecular techniques. There is a wealth of literature describing new antibodies and molecular tests and panels, but it can be especially overwhelming to decipher which of these publications are not biased by a manufacturer, and which antibodies,

molecular tests, or combination of tests are actually most practical in the workup of a specific neoplasm or clinical presentation. For this reason, the major focus in this issue was not a mere listing of commercially available ancillary tests or those cited in the literature, but rather the efficient utilization of these ancillary tests based on differential diagnoses generated by the cytologic examination. Although the authors review the literature, more importantly, they cite which of these tests are most practical. This approach is of critical importance, especially because we need to be more conservative in handling an already limited cytology sample, and knowledgeable of the most efficient way to triage a specimen.

In this timely review we gathered some of the top experts in their fields to discuss the utilization of ancillary studies in cytologic specimens. The topics covered include pancreas, lung, thyroid, salivary glands, urine, gynecologic Pap tests, and metastases of unknown origin. We followed a unique outline, beginning with an introductory overview and cytologic description emphasizing differential diagnosis, followed by review of ancillary tests being used in the diagnosis of disease, and those that have therapeutic and prognostic applications. In the "practical applications" sections, the authors discuss which of those tests are best used, based on their expert opinions and review of the literature. Each article ends with a brief summary of "future trends": what the authors think is coming down the pipeline that may further reform our practice, especially as it relates to molecular testing. For easy and quick

Surgical Pathology 7 (2014) ix–x
http://dx.doi.org/10.1016/j.path.2014.01.001
1875-9181/14/$ – see front matter © 2014 Elsevier Inc. All rights reserved.

reference, many boxes and tables are inserted throughout the text emphasizing key points, differential diagnosis, and potential pitfalls associated with interpretation of ancillary results.

Finally, I would like to declare that my involvement in this publication has been an absolute pleasure, especially working with all the authors and seeing their outstanding contributions come to fruition. I would like to give special thanks to Dr John Goldblum for inviting me to be a guest editor, and to Joanne Husovski for her excellent organizing skills and seeing this project to completion. Last but not least, I would like to thank the special people in my life for their love and support, including my parents; my kids, Omar, Nour, and Deena; and my girlfriend, Angie.

Tarik M. Elsheikh, MD
Medical Director of Anatomic Pathology Services
Cleveland Clinic Laboratories Cleveland, Ohio

E-mail address:
elsheit@ccf.org

Ancillary Studies, Including Immunohistochemistry and Molecular Studies, in Pancreatic Cytology

Michelle D. Reid, MD, MS[a], Barbara A. Centeno, MD[b],*

KEYWORDS

• Ancillary studies • Fine-needle aspiration • Pancreas

ABSTRACT

Fine-needle aspiration biopsy of the pancreas is indicated for sampling of solid and cystic masses. Preoperative cytologic diagnosis of pancreatic ductal adenocarcinoma and cystic lesions on cytology can be problematic, and ancillary studies may help confirm diagnosis. Ancillary studies in pancreatic cytology include special stains, immunohistochemistry, mutational analyses of specific genes, cyst fluid analysis of tumor markers and enzymes, and, in some instances, flow cytometry. Proteomics, microRNA sequencing, and whole-exome gene sequencing have been used to illustrate the progression of pancreatic neoplasms and identify key diagnostic markers. This article summarizes recent literature on ancillary studies in pancreatic fine-needle aspiration samples.

OVERVIEW

Fine-needle aspiration biopsy (FNAB) is the most effective procedure for sampling solid and cystic masses of the pancreas. Guidance techniques include intraoperative palpation and direct visualization, CT, and ultrasound, including endoscopic ultrasound (EUS).

An integrative approach to the evaluation of pancreatic aspirates, incorporating the clinical history, radiologic findings, cytologic findings, and ancillary studies, yields the most clinically relevant interpretation of aspirate material. The most crucial of these are imaging findings indicating whether a suspicious lesion is solid or cystic, because this information determines the cytopathologic algorithm. Different diagnostic entities are considered depending on whether the imaging studies show a mass that is solid, mixed solid and cystic, purely cystic, or cystic with a connection to the ductal system (an intraductal lesion).

ANCILLARY STUDIES

Ancillary studies available for use with pancreatic FNAB include histochemical stains, immunohistochemistry (IHC), flow cytometry, and cyst fluid analysis for enzymes, tumor markers, and mutational analyses. Ancillary studies are used most routinely for the differential diagnosis of nonductal solid neoplasms and metastases and the work-up of pancreatic cyst fluids.

[a] Department of Pathology, Emory University Hospital, Room H189, 1364 Clifton Road, NE, Atlanta, GA 30322, USA; [b] H. Lee Moffitt Cancer Center and Research Institute, 12902 Magnolia Drive, MCC 2071H, Tampa, FL 33612, USA
* Corresponding author.
E-mail address: Barbara.Centeno@moffitt.org

Surgical Pathology 7 (2014) 1–34
http://dx.doi.org/10.1016/j.path.2013.11.001
1875-9181/14/$ – see front matter © 2014 Elsevier Inc. All rights reserved.

ANCILLARY STUDIES IN SOLID PANCREATIC NEOPLASMS

Histochemical Stains

The use of special stains in the cytologic diagnosis of solid pancreatic neoplasms is somewhat limited and has been superseded by IHC. In tumors with ductal differentiation, including pancreatic ductal adenocarcinoma (PDA), intracytoplasmic mucin can be demonstrated with mucicarmine and periodic acid–Schiff (PAS) stains. PAS stain with diastase has also been helpful in diagnosing acinar cell carcinoma and solid pseudopapillary neoplasm (SPN). In acinar cell carcinoma, PAS-positive, diastase-resistant staining occurs in cytoplasmic zymogen granules, and in SPN, PAS-positive, diastase-resistant globules are seen in both cytoplasm and extracellular environ. Not all acinar cell carcinomas contain zymogen granules, however, making the diagnostic utility of PAS limited.

Immunohistochemistry

IHC studies have proven useful in the cytologic diagnosis of solid tumors. For PDA and its variants, ductal differentiation is supported by tumor positivity for carbohydrate cancer antigen (CA19-9), carcinoembryonic antigen (CEA), MUC1, cytokeratin (CK) 7, and CK19. Distinction of PDA from reactive ductal cells in chronic pancreatitis can be challenging on cytomorphology, and IHC can help distinguish the two. PDA is positive for p53 and negative or weakly positive for caudal-related homeobox 2 (CDX2) and often shows loss of deleted in pancreatic cancer (Dpc4) protein. In addition, PDA is positive for maspin, S100P, and insulin-like growth factor 2 mRNA-binding protein 3 (IMP-3) and negative for von Hippel-Lindau protein (pVHL), whereas reactive ductal cells show opposite results.[1] IHC markers of neuroendocrine differentiation include synaptophysin, chromogranin A, CD56, and CD57. In addition, some neuroendocrine tumors are positive for CK19, which is associated with more aggressive behavior. The ki-67 immunostain is critical for the grading of neuroendocrine neoplasms, through calculation of the ki-67 labeling index.[2] Markers of acinar differentiation include pancreatic enzymes trypsin and chymotrypsin. These are positive in acinar cell carcinoma and pancreatoblastomas with acinar differentiation. BCL10 is an additional marker of acinar cell carcinoma.[3] For mixed acinar-neuroendocrine carcinomas, tumor cells express both acinar and neuroendocrine markers. SPNs are of uncertain lineage with no normal equivalent in the non-neoplastic pancreas.

These tumors show a unique immunoprofile and are negative or focally positive for pancytokeratin but stain positively for β-catenin (nuclear expression), CD10, vimentin, and progesterone receptor (PR).

Molecular Studies

Molecular testing has been used more recently in the diagnosis of multiple solid pancreatic neoplasms. Whole-exome sequencing in PDA has demonstrated somatic mutations in key driver genes, KRAS, p16/CDKN2A, DPC4/SMAD4, and TP53. MicroRNA (miRNA) sequencing has also shown alterations in PDA resections and needle aspirates.[4] These involve many miRNAs, including miR-21, miR-155, miR-221,[5] miR-200c, and miR-451,[4] to name a few. Molecular analysis of pancreatic neuroendocrine tumors has demonstrated somatic mutations of death domain–associated protein (DAXX) and α-thalassemia/mental retardation syndrome X-linked (ATRX) genes, which result in loss of IHC expression of DAXX and ATRX proteins in tumor cells.[6] Chromosomal studies have revealed numerous complex karyotypes in acinar cell carcinoma, including aneuploidy, loss of chromosome 11p, and mutations in the APC/β-catenin gene.

Flow Cytometry

Flow cytometry typically is not used in the diagnosis of solid pancreatic tumors. However because lymphomas[7] and plasmacytomas may, involve the pancreas[8] and may resemble well-differentiated pancreatic neuroendocrine tumors (PanNETs), flow cytometry may play a critical role in distinguishing these differentials, by demonstrating clonal plasma cell or lymphoid populations.

CYTOLOGIC AND ANCILLARY FINDINGS IN SOLID PANCREATIC NEOPLASMS

PANCREATIC DUCTAL ADENOCARCINOMA

PDA accounts for 85% of solid pancreatic tumors. The cytologic diagnosis of poorly differentiated PDA is not typically a diagnostic challenge because neoplastic cells show overt malignant features (Fig. 1).[9,10] Well-differentiated PDA is more challenging because the cytologic features are subtle and easily misinterpreted as benign or reactive cells of chronic pancreatitis. The most characteristic cytologic findings in well-differentiated PDA are poorly formed ductal sheets with focal nuclear crowding (so-called "drunken" honeycomb sheets) (Fig. 2),[9,10] with only minimal deviation from normal duct morphology.

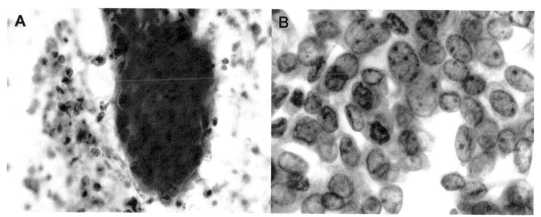

Fig. 1. Poorly differentiated PDA. Neoplastic cells are arranged in (*A*) 3-D clusters and show marked nuclear pleomorphism and irregular hyperchromatic nuclei with prominent macronucleoli (Papanicolaou stain, ×400 magnification). (*B*) Tumor cells are arranged in a flat sheet, show obvious malignant features and nuclear hypochromasia (Papanicolaou stain, ×400 magnification).

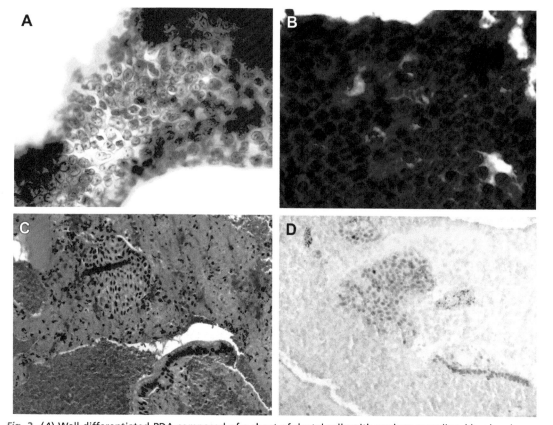

Fig. 2. (*A*) Well-differentiated PDA composed of a sheet of ductal cells with nuclear crowding (drunken honeycomb) and nuclear membrane irregularity (Papanicolaou stain, ×400 magnification). (*B*) Reactive ductal cells are also arranged in a flat sheet with evenly spaced nuclei with rounded borders and slight nuclear enlargement (Papanicolaou stain, ×400 magnification). (*C*) Cellblock section showing cluster of well-differentiated PDA tumor cells on the upper left and a strip of benign gastric epithelium at the lower right (hematoxylin-eosin stain, ×200 magnification). (*D*) Tumor cells are focally positive for p53 immunostain whereas gastric epithelium is negative (magnification ×200).

Ancillary Studies in the Diagnosis of Pancreatic Ductal Adenocarcinoma

Immunohistochemistry

Somatic mutations of the *TP53* gene result in nuclear staining of PDA tumor cells with the p53 immunostain,[11] which is negative in reactive ductal cells.[12–15] CDX2 is negative or weakly positive in PDA and negative in reactive ductal cells. Somatic inactivation of the *DPC4/SMAD4* gene (which occurs in approximately half of PDAs) results in loss of Dpc4 staining in PDA[1,13–15] whereas Dpc4 is positive or preserved in reactive ductal cells.[12]

A panel of antibodies combining pVHL, maspin, S100P, and IMP-3 is effective in distinguishing PDA from reactive pancreatic ductal cells.[1] Most (>90%) PDAs are positive for maspin, S100P, and IMP-3 and negative for pVHL, in contrast to reactive ductal cells, which are positive for pVHL and typically negative for IMP-3, maspin, and S100P. A limitation of maspin and S100P, however, is that they may be positive in gastric and duodenal epithelial contaminants, which limits their sensitivity in EUS-guided fine-needle aspirations (FNAs), in which these contaminants are frequent. p53 Is negative in gastrointestinal tract (GIT) contaminants (duodenal and gastric epithelium) but positive in PDA (see **Fig. 2**), and, unlike PDA, reactive ductal cells and GIT contaminants retain Dpc4.[13,15]

Molecular testing

Somatic mutations of the *KRAS* oncogene and the tumor suppressor genes, *p16/CDKN2A*, *DPC4/SMAD4*, and *TP53*, are often seen in PDA.[13,15] Pyrosequencing performed on microdissected cellblock material may identify these *KRAS* mutations, which occur in more than 90% of PDAs.[16] Such mutations are not present in reactive ductal cells or GIT contaminants. miRNA alterations in miR-21, miR-155, and miR-221 occur in PDA.[5] miRNA sequencing of microdissected tumor cells from formalin-fixed paraffin-embedded cellblock material has been used to identify these alterations.[4]

Key Points
PANCREATIC DUCTAL ADENOCARCINOMA

1. Most common solid pancreatic tumor.

2. Well-differentiated carcinoma may resemble reactive ductal cells and GIT epithelial contaminants.

3. Diagnosis is supported by
   - Tumor cell positivity for p53, maspin, S100P, and IMP-3 and negativity for Dpc4 and pVHL.
   - IHC panel combining p53 and Dpc4 is useful in distinguishing PDA from reactive ductal cells.
   - *KRAS* and *p16/CDKN2A* mutation.

Differential Diagnosis
OF PANCREATIC DUCTAL ADENOCARCINOMA

1. Reactive ductal cells in chronic pancreatitis
   - Reactive ductal cells are arranged as honeycomb sheets with minimal cytologic atypia.
   - Reactive ductal cells are negative for p53, maspin, S100P, and IMP-3 and positive for Dpc4 and pVHL.
   - PDA is positive for p53, maspin, S100P, and IMP-3; negative for Dpc4 and pVHL; and negative or focally positive for CDX2.
   - PDA shows somatic mutations of *K-RAS*, *p16/CDKN2A*, *p53*, and *DPC4/SMAD4*, which are not seen in reactive ductal cells.

2. GIT epithelial contaminants
   - Duodenal epithelium forms sheets of columnar cells with interspersed goblet cells and has an associated brush border.[9,17]
   - Duodenal epithelium is positive for CDX2 and Dpc4 but negative for p53 immunostain.
   - Duodenal and gastric epithelium may stain with maspin and S100P.
   - Mutations of *KRAS*, *p16/CDKN2A*, *p53*, and *DPC4/SMAD4* are not seen in GIT epithelium.

PANCREATIC NEUROENDOCRINE NEOPLASMS

Pancreatic neuroendocrine neoplasms are typically solid tumors and account for 4% of all pancreatic tumors. Most occur in adults but may rarely be seen in children. In 2010, the World Health Organization modified their classification to include 3 grades and 2 levels of differentiation (well-differentiated PanNETs [grade 1 and 2 tumors] and poorly differentiated neuroendocrine carcinoma [grade 3 tumors]).[18] This grading system correlates strongly with clinical outcome.[18,19] Grading is based on morphology and proliferative activity, the latter being a combined assessment of mitoses per 10 high-power fields (HPFs), after counting 50 HPFs, and the ki-67 index/500–2000 tumor cells (Table 1).

In well-differentiated PanNETs, neoplastic cells are typically small to intermediate, singly dispersed or clustered with oval nuclei, salt-and-pepper chromatin, and plasmacytoid cytomorphology (Fig. 3).[9,10] Rosette-like structures with central fibrovascular cores may also be seen (see Fig. 3).[20,21] In poorly differentiated (grade 3) small

Table 1
Grading of pancreatic neuroendocrine neoplasms

	Well-Differentiated PanNET		Poorly-Differentiated PanNEC
	Grade 1	Grade 2	Grade 3
Mitotic count	<2/10 HPF	2–20/10 HPF	>20/10 HPF
ki-67 index (%)	<3	3–20	>20

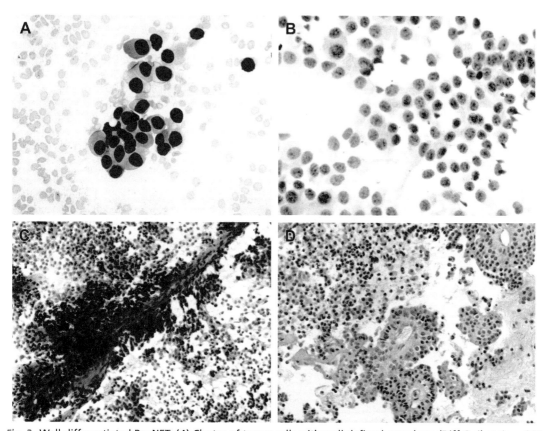

Fig. 3. Well-differentiated PanNET. (A) Cluster of tumor cells with well-defined cytoplasm (Diff-Quik stain, ×200 magnification). (B) Tumor cells are dispersed as dishesive plasmacytoid cells with dense cytoplasm and salt-and-pepper chromatin (Papanicolaou stain, ×400 magnification). (C) A rosette-like structure is visible on smear and has a central fibrovascular core with crowded but dishesive tumor cells surrounding it (Papanicolaou stain, ×200 magnification). (D) Numerous rosettes are present on the cellblock section of a PanNET (hematoxylin-eosin stain, ×200 magnification).

cell or large cell neuroendocrine carcinoma, the tumor cells are small or large and show malignant features (**Fig. 4**).[20]

Ancillary Studies in the Diagnosis of Pancreatic Neuroendocrine Neoplasms

Immunohistochemistry

A diagnosis of pancreatic neuroendocrine tumor (PanNET) or pancreatic neuroendocrine carcinoma (PanNEC) is supported by tumor cell expression of neuroendocrine markers (synaptophysin, chromogranin A, CD56, and CD57) as well as pancytokeratin (**Fig. 5**).[21,22] Ki-67 staining is useful in tumor grading.[2,23,24] Pancreatic neuroendocrine neoplasms may resemble lymphoma on cytology (see **Fig. 4**) but the two can be distinguished by IHC because neuroendocrine neoplasms are pancytokeratin positive and express neuroendocrine markers whereas lymphoma is negative for pancytokeratin and neuroendocrine markers but positive for leukocyte common antigen (LCA).

Plasmacytomas may arise in the pancreas and can be difficult to distinguish cytologically from neuroendocrine tumors with prominent plasmacytoid features.[8] Plasmacytomas, however, express CD138 and are negative for pancytokeratin. In addition, CD38 expression and κ or λ light chain restriction on flow cytometry favor plasmacytoma over PanNET. The importance of specimen triage at the time of immediate evaluation cannot be overstated in such situations. If lymphoma or plasmacytoma is suspected at the time of on-site evaluation, a sample should be collected in RPMI medium and submitted for flow cytometry.

SPNs may contain the fibrovascular cores typically seen in PanNETs. Additionally, SPNs may express the neuroendocrine markers, CD56 and synaptophysin, but synaptophysin staining is often focal. In addition, SPNs are usually pancytokeratin negative (or only focally positive) and show strong nuclear positivity for β-catenin as well as PR and vimentin, whereas PanNETs are typically negative for these markers.

Acinar cell carcinomas may resemble PanNETs cytologically, but they are usually trypsin and chymotrypsin positive whereas these stains are negative in PanNETs.

Molecular studies

Molecular studies in PanNETs revealed somatic mutations of the *DAXX* and *ATRX* genes, which are involved in chromatin remodeling and telomere maintenance.[6,25,26] As a result, these tumors may also show loss of expression of DAXX and ATRX IHC proteins.[6] *Rb* and *TP53* gene mutations have been identified in PanNEC but not in well-differentiated PanNET. BCL2 protein is also overexpressed in PDNEC (100% of small cell carcinoma and 50% of large cell carcinomas) but is negative or focally positive in well-differentiated PanNET.[27]

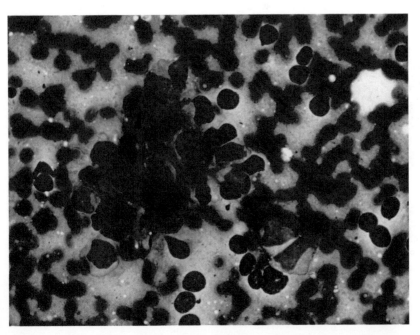

Fig. 4. Poorly differentiated small cell neuroendocrine carcinoma. Tumor cells are disposed as clusters of small cells with scant cytoplasm and focal nuclear molding (Diff-Quik stain, ×400 magnification).

ACINAR CELL CARCINOMA

Acinar cell carcinoma is a rare solid, stroma-poor primary pancreatic tumor of acinar lineage. Most tumors arise in older adults but may rarely be seen in children. Smears are hypercellular and composed of sheets and clusters or singly dispersed epithelial cells with zymogen-rich, granular cytoplasm (**Fig. 6**). Nuclei are round to oval with fine to coarse chromatin and prominent nucleoli.[21,28] These tumors are also notoriously mitotically active. Although the cytologic features of acinar cell carcinoma are thought to be distinctive some investigators have shown that these tumors can be misdiagnosed on cytology.[29]

Ancillary Studies in the Diagnosis of Acinar Cell Carcinoma

Immunohistochemistry
Immunocytochemistry is critical to the accurate diagnosis of acinar cell carcinoma because tumor

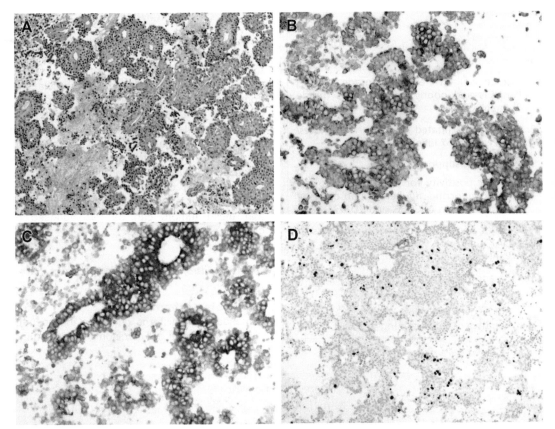

Fig. 5. Well-differentiated PanNET. (*A*) Cellblock section shows numerous rosettes (hematoxylin-eosin stain, ×200 magnification). Tumor cells are strongly and diffusely positive for (*B*) pancytokeratin and (*C*) synaptophysin and (*D*) are focally positive for ki-67 (×200 magnification). In this example, the ki-67 index was 8%, consistent with a grade 2 well-differentiated PanNET.

cells resemble normal pancreatic acini as well as other pancreatic tumors. Unfortunately, immuno-chemical distinction between normal acinar cells and tumor cells of acinar cell carcinoma is not possible. On cytology, however, normal pancreatic acinar cells are small and typically arranged in grapelike clusters or acini with central lumina. In acinar cell carcinoma, smears are more hypercellular with clusters and syncytial aggregates of large epithelial cells with prominent nucleoli and brisk mitotic activity. Acinar cell carcinoma stains positively for pancytokeratin and variably expresses pancreatic enzymes amylase, lipase, elastase, and phospholipase 2.[9,21] The most sensitive IHC marker for acinar cell carcinoma is trypsin, which diffusely stains tumor cells (see **Fig. 6**).[29] BCL10 is also positive in more than 80% of tumors, including trypsin-negative

tumors.[3] The BCL10 antibody is directed against the COOH-terminal portion of BCL10 protein, which recognizes the COOH-terminal portion of carboxyl ester lipase (CEL). PAS may also stain cytoplasmic zymogen granules.

Acinar cell carcinoma may resemble pancreatic neuroendocrine neoplasms because of their similarity in cell size and abundant singly dispersed cells.[21] Another noteworthy differential is mixed acinar-neuroendocrine carcinoma, in which, by definition, more than 30% of tumor cells show neuroendocrine differentiation.[30] This acinar cell neoplasm can be diagnosed on cytologic samples based on mixed cytomorphology as well as expression of both acinar and neuroendocrine IHC markers (**Fig. 7**).[29]

Another diagnostic differential is pancreatoblastoma. This tumor often shows focal or diffuse

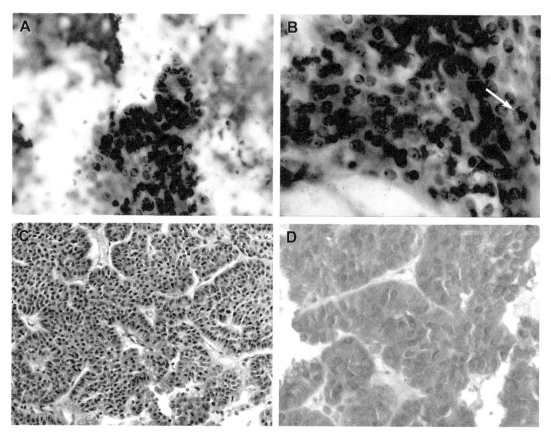

Fig. 6. Acinar cell carcinoma. (*A*) The smear shows tumor cells with abundant granular cytoplasm forming clusters and focal acinar structures (Papanicolaou stain ×200 magnification). (*B*) A Papanicolaou-stained smear shows syncytial groups of cells with large vesicular nuclei, prominent macronucleoli, and abnormal mitotic figures (*arrow*) (×400 magnification). (*C*) Cellblock section is hypercellular and shows anastomosing trabeculae and sheets of stroma-poor epithelial cells (hematoxylin-eosin stain, ×200 magnification). (*D*) Tumor cells show diffuse cytoplasmic positivity for trypsin immunostain (magnification ×400).

acinar differentiation and stains positively for trypsin, chymotrypsin, and lipase. Distinction from acinar cell carcinoma may be extremely difficult without the identification of primitive (blastemal), mesenchymal elements, or squamoid morules. The latter are difficult to identify, however, on cytologic smears and if seen are usually present on cellblock sections.[31,32]

Molecular studies

Acinar cell carcinomas may harbor allelic loss on chromosome 11p and approximately a fourth of the cases have shown mutations in *APC*/β-catenin.[33] The PDA-related genetic mutations and their associated IHC profiles (*KRAS*, *p16/CDKN2A*, *p53*, and *DPC4/SMAD4*) are not described in acinar cell carcinoma.[15] The mutations in pancreatic neuroendocrine tumors (*DAXX/ATRX*) have also not been described in acinar cell carcinoma,[11] which may be helpful in differentiating the two.

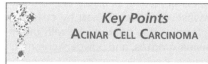

Key Points
ACINAR CELL CARCINOMA

1. Tumor cells stain positively for pancytokeratin, trypsin, chymotrypsin, and BCL10.

2. Positivity for PAS (with diastase resistance) may be seen in some cases.

Differential Diagnosis
OF ACINAR CELL CARCINOMA

1. Benign acinar cells
   - Cells are arranged as grapelike clusters of bland epithelial cells with individual acini containing central lumina.
   - Immunohistochemistry is not useful in the distinction of benign acinar cells from acinar cell carcinoma.

2. PanNET
   - Tumor cells may be similar in appearance to acinar cell carcinoma; however, nuclei contain salt-and-pepper chromatin.
   - PanNETs express neuroendocrine markers but are negative for trypsin and chymotrypsin.
   - Acinar cell carcinoma is positive for trypsin and chymotrypsin, and negative for neuroendocrine markers.

3. Mixed acinar-neuroendocrine carcinoma.
   - Cytomorphology may show a mixed population of acinar and neuroendocrine-type cells.
   - Both neuroendocrine and acinar markers should be performed to facilitate accurate diagnosis.
   - Tumor cells express both acinar (trypsin and chymotrypsin) and neuroendocrine markers.

4. Pancreatoblastoma
   - Cytologic distinction may be impossible because both tumors stain with markers of acinar differentiation.
   - Identification of blastemal, mesenchymal elements, or squamoid morules is helpful.
   - Unfortunately squamoid morules are only rarely seen on cytologic samples.

SOLID PSEUDOPAPILLARY NEOPLASM

SPNs are rare low-grade pancreatic neoplasms that account for 3% of all pancreatic tumors. Tumors typically arise in young patients in the second or third decade and show a strong female preponderance and a propensity for involvement of the pancreatic tail.[9]

Their cytomorphology is distinct, making the diagnosis highly specific on aspiration.[34,35] Cytology yields branching papillary clusters with central fibrovascular cores,[34] lined by cells with scant cytoplasm, coffee bean nuclei with prominent longitudinal grooves, and powdery chromatin (Fig. 8). Because of cytoplasmic fragility, smearing often results in numerous naked bean–shaped nuclei in the smear background. On Diff-Quik stain, the fibrovascular cores are often surrounded by a myxoid magenta-colored stroma (see Fig. 8).[36]

Ancillary Studies in the Diagnosis of Solid Pseudopapillary Neoplasm

Immunohistochemistry and molecular studies

Tumor cells in SPN are typically negative or only focally positive for pancytokeratin and strongly express nuclear β-catenin in most cases.[15] β-Catenin expression is due to activating somatic mutations in the β-catenin gene (CTNNB1), which occurs in more than 90% of cases,[37,38] and results in nuclear accumulation of β-catenin protein (Fig. 9). Mutations in CTNNB1 also cause aberrant E-cadherin expression in tumor nuclei, which may explain the characteristic discohesion often seen in these tumors.[39] SPNs also express CD10, CD56, PR, and vimentin.[9,10,34]

A key cytologic differential for SPN is a well-differentiated PanNET, which may also show branching clusters with fibrovascular cores and

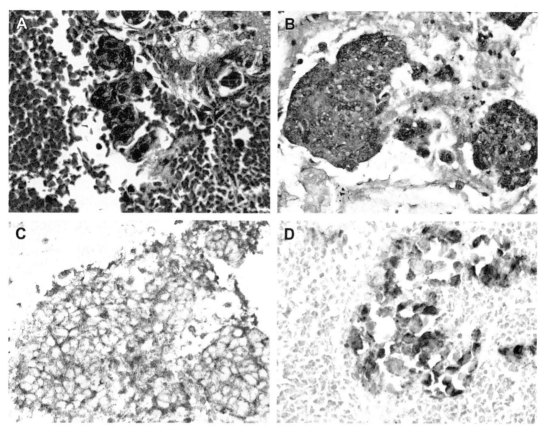

Fig. 7. Mixed acinar-neuroendocrine carcinoma. (*A*) Cellblock section shows clusters of malignant tumor cells with prominent nucleoli and background necrosis (hematoxylin-eosin stain, ×600 magnification). (*B*) Tumor cells are positive for PAS stain (magnification ×400), (*C*) synaptophysin (magnification ×400), and (*D*) trypsin (magnification ×400).

single cells. PanNETs, however, are diffusely and strongly positive for pancytokeratin and neuroendocrine markers, whereas SPNs only rarely and focally express pancytokeratin and are negative - or only focally positive for neuroendocrine markers.

Serous cystadenomas (SCAs) and neoplastic mucinous cysts (NMCs) may resemble SPNs on imaging. SCAs usually result, however, in hypocellular smears with rare low cuboidal to columnar cells lacking the longitudinal nuclear grooves typical of SPNs. SCAs are diffusely positive for pancytokeratin and PAS whereas SPNs are not. NMCs have thick background mucin and pancytokeratin-positive mucin-rich epithelial cells on smears, which are not seen in SPNs.

Key Points
SOLID PSEUDOPAPILLARY NEOPLASM

1. Rare low-grade malignant neoplasm of uncertain lineage.

2. Cytologic features are distinctive.

3. Diagnosis is supported by

   - Tumor cell positivity for β-catenin (nuclear), CD10, vimentin, and PR and negativity or focal staining for pancytokeratin.

   - Tumor cells may express neuroendocrine markers CD56 and synaptophysin.

   - Somatic mutations in *CTNNB1* occur in most cases.

Solid pancreatic neoplasms

1. PanNET, well differentiated

   - May have branching papillae or rosettes similar to SPNs.

   - Tumor cells have salt-and-pepper chromatin, unlike the powdery chromatin in SPNs.

   - PanNETs are positive for pancytokeratin and neuroendocrine markers and negative for β-catenin, CD10, PR, and vimentin.

   - PanNETs also show loss of DAXX and ATRX proteins on IHC.

Cystic pancreatic neoplasms

1. SCA

   - Smears are typically paucicellular, with cells showing clear cytoplasm, that stain diffusely for pancytokeratin, unlike SPNs.

2. NMCs (intraductal papillary mucinous neoplasm [IPMN] and mucinous cystic neoplasm [MCN])

   - Smear background contains thick colloid-like mucin and mucin-rich epithelial cells.

   - Tumor cells are negative for β-catenin, CD10, PR, and vimentin and positive for pancytokeratin and mucicarmine.

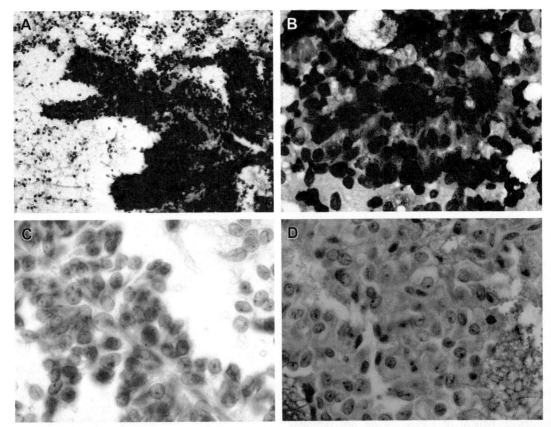

Fig. 8. SPN. (*A*) Hypercellular smear composed of branching, finger-like papillae with surrounding singly dispersed naked nuclei (Papanicolaou stain, ×100 magnification). (*B*) Cluster of tumor cells with vague papillary outline is intimately admixed with magenta-colored myxoid stroma (Diff-Quik stain, ×400 magnification). (*C*) Distinct fibrovascular cores are lined by bland-appearing cells with scant cytoplasm and vesicular nuclei with longitudinal nuclear grooves (Papanicolaou stain, ×400 magnification). (*D*) Cellblock section shows sheet of stroma-poor epithelioid cells with vesicular nuclei and prominent nuclear grooves (Papanicolaou stain, ×400 magnification).

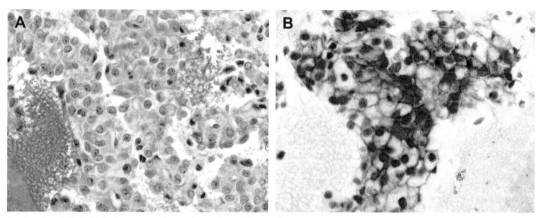

Fig. 9. SPN. (*A*) Cellblock section shows branching sheet of tumor cells (Papanicolaou stain, ×200 magnification), with (*B*) nuclear positivity for β-catenin (×200 magnification).

PANCREATOBLASTOMA

Pancreatoblastoma, an extremely rare malignant trilineage neoplasm, is most commonly seen in the pediatric population. One-third of tumors, however, occur in adults. Smears are usually hypercellular and often show neoplastic cells with acinar differentiation.[31,40] In addition, they may show ductal, neuroendocrine, and mesenchymal components on cytologic specimens.[31,32,40] The squamoid morules, which are a characteristic histologic feature, are not typically seen in cytologic specimens, except rarely on cellblock or ultrastructural examination.[9,31,32,40]

Ancillary Studies in the Diagnosis of Pancreatoblastoma

Immunohistochemistry
The IHC profile of pancreatoblastoma is dependent on the line of differentiation of tumor cells. The acinar component may be PAS positive and express trypsin, lipase, and chymotrypsin. The squamoid morules are composed of biotin-rich optically clear nuclei (BROCN), which may overexpress estrogen receptor β and β-catenin (both nuclear and cytoplasmic).[41] Unfortunately, because they are rarely seen in cytologic samples, they are unlikely to be helpful in cytologic diagnosis.

Because of acinar differentiation, pancreatoblastomas must be distinguished from acinar cell carcinoma on cytology. IHC, however, is unlikely to be helpful in this distinction, because both tumors express markers of acinar differentiation. In such situations, clinical information is especially critical, and in some cases final classification may have to be deferred to excision. The presence of a variety of different cell types within the same tumor (including neuroendocrine as well as primitive or mesenchymal-type cells) may aid in classification.

Key Points
PANCREATOBLASTOMA

1. Cytomorphologically and immunophenotypically similar to acinar cell carcinoma (trypsin and chymotrypsin positive).

2. Diagnosis is supported by identification of squamoid morules, but these are rarely seen on cytology.

Differential Diagnosis
OF PANCREATOBLASTOMA

Acinar cell carcinoma

- Tumor cells may appear similar to pancreatoblastomas with extensive acinar differentiation.

- The presence of nonacinar (ductal, mesenchymal, and primitive) elements distinguishes pancreatoblastoma from acinar cell carcinoma, which lacks these elements.

- IHC may not be helpful in distinction because the two may show similar acinar immunoprofile.

- Lacks squamoid morules.

SECONDARY PANCREATIC NEOPLASMS

Many tumors may secondarily involve the pancreas both on surgical and cytologic samples.[7,42,43] Studies have recently shown that the most common secondary tumor to involve the pancreas is renal cell carcinoma.[7,43] The biggest clue to diagnosing metastases is to recognize cytology that is foreign to the pancreas (ie, the malignant cells do not have cytologic features of the more common primary pancreatic tumors, such as PDA and acinar and neuroendocrine carcinoma). Other tumors that may metastasize to the pancreas include lung carcinoma (small cell carcinoma, adenocarcinoma, and squamous cell carcinoma), breast carcinoma, melanoma, and sarcoma as well as lymphoma.[7,43] Clinical history of previous malignancy is critical to cytologic diagnosis, so too is the performance of key differentiating IHC panels in suspicious cases. Accurate cytologic diagnosis of metastatic disease involving the pancreas is important because it can prevent unnecessary surgery. However it has been shown that in some tumors pancreatectomy improves patient outcome.[44]

Key Points
SECONDARY PANCREATIC NEOPLASMS

1. Most common secondary tumor is renal cell carcinoma.

2. History of prior malignancy facilitates accurate diagnosis and selection of appropriate IHC panels.

3. Cytology foreign to the pancreas is the biggest clue.

ANCILLARY STUDIES IN CYSTIC MASSES

The most significant entities included in the differential diagnosis of cystic lesions include pseudocyst, non-neoplastic cysts, and neoplastic cysts. Neoplastic cysts include SCA, solid neoplasms that have undergone cystic degeneration, IPMN, and MCN.

Pancreatic cyst fluid analysis incorporates gross examination of the fluid, cytology, and ancillary studies, including viscosity measurements, enzyme and tumor marker levels, and mutational analysis. Most of the biochemical and molecular testing is performed on an aliquot of cyst fluid, which can be diluted, and the value compensated by the amount of dilution.[45] Theoretically, the supernatant of the fluid provides sufficient material for CEA and amylase analysis and adequate DNA for molecular analysis. Special stains and IHC may be performed on the corresponding cytology specimens if applicable. Patient management is based on correlation of cytology findings, ancillary studies, imaging, and clinical findings.

Viscosity

Initial studies used viscosity measurements to distinguish between nonmucinous and mucinous lesions.[45] Viscosity levels greater than serum correlated with mucinous cysts. False-positive results, however, resulted from other cysts with thick, luminal contents, such as lymphoepithelial cysts of the pancreas (LECPs),[46] and other lesions with viscous or mucinous contents. A recent study emphasized again the value of assessing the viscosity of the fluid.[47] In this study, viscosity was determined by an endosonographer placing a drop of fluid between the thumb and index finger and measuring the maximum length of stretch before disruption of the mucus string.

Enzymes

The measurement of amylase and lipase levels is helpful in differentiating pseudocysts from cystic neoplasms, such as SCA and MCN. Amylase isoenzyme analysis provided even more specific information, but this technique did not gain popularity.[45] Currently, only amylase levels are measured in pancreatic cyst fluids.

Key Points
CYST FLUID AMYLASE LEVELS

1. Elevated in inflammatory processes and lesions with a connection to the ductal system.

2. Hemorrhagic or cystic degeneration may lead to spuriously elevated levels in SCA.

Tumor Markers

Many tumor markers have been evaluated and reported on in the literature for the evaluation of pancreatic cysts,[45] but, currently, CEA is the only one measured routinely. Elevated CEA is seen in both non-neoplastic and neoplastic cystic lesions with mucin but also in some nonmucinous cysts, including mesothelial inclusion cysts and LECPs. A cutoff level of 192 ng/mL was established as indicative of a mucinous-type neoplasm (MCN or IPMN)[48]; however, lower levels do not exclude the diagnosis. Although CA19-9 remains a useful serum tumor marker to monitor pancreatic carcinoma, it is not useful in pancreatic cyst fluids because its levels are highly variable and unreliable.[45]

Histochemical Stains

Mucicarmine stain and PAS with and without diastase may be used for the identification of mucin and glycogen, respectively. The utility of special stains in cyst fluid samples is, however, limited.

Immunohistochemistry

The role of IHC in the work-up of cystic lesions is most often for the differential diagnosis of solid neoplasms that have undergone cystic degeneration, such as PanNET and SPN, or for the differential diagnosis of nonmucinous lesions and suspected metastases.

IHC may be used to identify specific types of IPMN epithelium and gastric and duodenal contaminants. Mutations associated with the usual PDA, such as *p53* and *SMAD4/DPC4*, are more variably detected in MCN and IPMN. When present, however, they can help diagnose PDA associated with IPMN/MCN.

Molecular Studies

KRAS

Analysis of pancreatic cyst fluid for *KRAS* gene mutations is useful in the distinction of NMCs (IPMN and MCN) from non-neoplastic cysts.[9,49–51] In one study, *KRAS* mutations were shown to have a sensitivity of 54% and a specificity of 100% for the detection of PDA, IPMN, and MCN. In the same study, cystic lesions with elevated CEA (including 1 retention cyst, 1 LECP, and 1 foregut cyst) lacked *KRAS* mutations. False-positive results, however, may occur in pseudocysts.[52] Sampling of pancreatic

intraepithelial neoplasia (PanIN) adjacent to a pseudocyst may account for some of the false-positive results (Centeno, personal communication). Somatic mutations seem more frequent in IPMN (67%) than in MCN (14%).[53]

GNAS

Recurrent mutations at codon 201 of the *GNAS* gene were identified in the cyst fluids of IPMN. These mutations were found in 66% of IPMNs studied and in seven of the eight invasive carcinomas developing from these *GNAS*-mutated IPMNs.[54] *GNAS* mutations were not identified in invasive carcinomas that were not associated with IPMNs, or in MCN and other neoplastic cysts.

DNA Analysis and Other Molecular Analysis

In addition to *KRAS* mutational analysis, measurement of pancreatic cyst fluid DNA quantity and quality and loss of heterozygosity (LOH) for 15 genomic loci associated with tumor suppressor genes has been incorporated into a commercially available assay, PathFinderTG (Redpath Integrated Pathology, Pittsburgh, Pennsylvania). Cysts are classified as mucinous, nonmucinous, or malignant based on DNA quantity and quality, *KRAS* gene point mutations, and the amplitude of *KRAS* and LOH mutations, when present. A limitation of PathFinderTG is that not all IPMNs or MCNs have *KRAS* mutations, thus resulting in false-negative results.

CYTOLOGIC AND ANCILLARY FEATURES OF CYSTIC MASSES

NON-NEOPLASTIC CYSTS

Pseudocyst

Pseudocysts are the most common cysts of the pancreas. Aspiration of a pseudocyst typically yields abundant turbid, brown fluid rich in hemosiderin-laden macrophages and few inflammatory cells, fibrin, debris, and bile pigment. Pseudocysts lack an epithelial lining (**Fig. 10**)[55,56] and do not contain mucin. Mucin, however, may be obtained as a contaminant from the GIT, resulting in a positive mucicarmine stain[57,58] and a false-positive diagnosis of mucinous cyst. Amylase levels are elevated in pseudocysts but CEA is low. *KRAS* and *GNAS* mutations are not present in pseudocysts.

Lymphoepithelial Cyst of the Pancreas

Lymphoepithelial cyst of the pancreas is a benign cyst with a male predominance. The cytology samples of LECPs usually yield a variable amount of pasty, yellow-gray, or yellow-white material.[59] Smears show abundant anucleated squames, keratinous debris, and few nucleated squamous cells with lymphocytes, histiocytes, background debris, cholesterol clefts, and crystals (**Fig. 11**).[60,61]

The lining epithelium of LECPs expresses CK7, CEA, CA19-9, MUC1, and MUC4 near the surface. P63 is expressed in the basal layer.[62] Squamous cells are negative for MUC5AC, MUC2, and MUC6. Mucous cells are seen in some LECPs, and these express MUC5AC and MUC4 but are negative for MUC1, MUC2, and MUC6. Cyst fluid CEA and amylase are elevated[46,62] but *KRAS* and *GNAS* mutations are not seen.

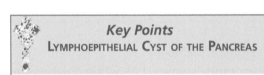

Key Points
LYMPHOEPITHELIAL CYST OF THE PANCREAS

1. Male predominance

2. Benign

3. Thick, pasty yellow-gray, or yellow-white material

4. Cytology shows anucleated squames, histiocyctes, cholesterol crystals, and granular layer; variable lymphocytes; and variable mucinous epithelium

5. CEA and amylase elevated

6. Lacks *KRAS* and *GNAS* mutations

Lymphoepithelial cyst of the pancreas	
Versus Differential Entity	**Distinguishing Feature(s) that Differ from Major Entity Under Discussion**
SCOPD	Thick background mucin, benign squamous epithelium lined by a glandular layer of epithelium, elevated CEA and amylase, MUC1+ glandular cells
Adenosquamous carcinoma	Malignant squamous and glandular component, CK5/6 and p63 positivity in squamous component, *KRAS* mutations
Metastatic squamous cell carcinoma	Malignant squamous cells, lacks mucinous component, CK5/6 and p63 positivity in squamous component
IPMN	Thick background mucin and glandular neoplastic cells, lacks squamous component, CEA and amylase elevated, *KRAS* and *GNAS* mutations
MCN	Thick background mucin, glandular neoplastic cells, lacks squamous component, CEA elevated, amylase low, *KRAS* mutations variably present.

Fig. 10. Pseudocyst. Cytospin showing histiocytes, background debris and pigment (Papanicolaou stain, 400 × magnification).

Fig. 11. LECP. (*A*) Degenerated squamous cells and cholesterol crystals (Diff-Quik, magnification ×200). (*B*) Cellblock showing anucleated squamous cells, and granular layer (Hematoxylin & Eosin stain, magnification ×400).

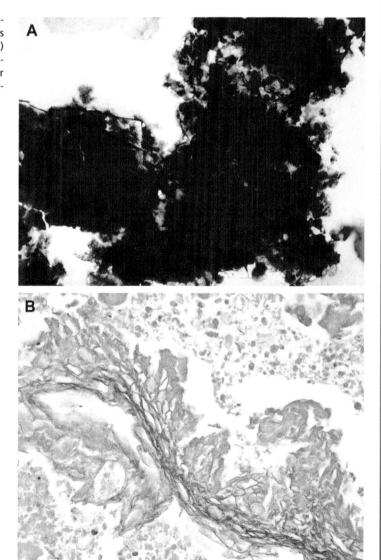

Squamoid Cyst of Pancreatic Ducts

Squamous cyst of pancreatic ducts (SCOPD) is a recently described entity that presents as a large cystic mass on imaging studies.[63] Cysts are lined by a layer of mucinous epithelium at the luminal surface, with an underlying layer of squamous epithelium at the base. Aspirates contain benign-appearing squamous cells, with benign mucinous columnar cells either surrounding the squamous epithelium or occurring separately.

Key Points
SQUAMOID CYST OF PANCREATIC DUCTS

1. Viscous, mucinous fluid.

2. Background mucin with histiocytes and oncotic cells.

3. Benign squamous cells, which may have a luminal layer of glandular epithelium.

4. Elevated CEA and amylase levels.

5. Special stains for mucin positive in glandular layer.

6. CK5/6 and p63 expressed in squamous layer, MUC1 in all layers.

The smear background is mucinous with oncotic cells.

IHC stains show positivity for CK5/6 and p63 in the squamous layer. The columnar, glandular layer contains intracytoplasmic mucin (positive mucicarmine stain). MUC1 is positive in both the squamous and glandular layers (**Fig. 12**). Cyst fluid analysis shows elevated CEA and amylase.

NEOPLASTIC CYSTS

Serous Cystadenoma

Aspiration of SCA typically yields scant clear, thin fluid. The background is watery, lacks thick mucin, and may contain fibrovascular stromal fragments stripped of epithelial cells. Cells are usually arranged in flat, monolayered sheets or as dispersed single cells or stripped nuclei, lacking nucleoli and mitoses (**Fig. 13**).[64] Aspirates may contain only a few cuboidal cells or histiocytes.[50] Because the stroma is typically quite vascular, these cysts may hemorrhage, leading to bloody smears with hemosiderin-laden macrophages.[50]

In SCA, the cytoplasm is clear due to glycogen, which can be demonstrated with PAS stains with and without diastase. Recently, GLUT1 has been identified as a marker of serous

Squamoid cyst of pancreatic ducts	
Versus Differential Entity	**Distinguishing Feature(s) that Differ from Major Entity Under Discussion**
1. Gastric epithelium	Honeycomb morphology, thinner mucin, no oncotic cells, low CEA, absence of *KRAS* and *GNAS* mutations
2. Small intestinal epithelium	Honeycomb morphology, goblet cells, lymphocytes, low CEA, absence of *KRAS* and *GNAS* mutations
3. LECP	Anucleated squames, debris, cholesterol crystals, lymphocytes may or may not be present, CEA and amylase elevated, lacks *KRAS* and *GNAS* mutations, MUC5AC and MUC4+ glandular cells
4. Retention cyst	Histiocytes, background mucin, may have ductal epithelium, CEA elevated, lacks *KRAS* mutations and *GNAS* mutations
5. IPMN	Connects to ductal system, glandular neoplastic epithelium no squamous cells, viscous fluid, elevated CEA, *KRAS* and *GNAS* mutations may be present
6. IOPN	Connects to ductal system, same background, oncocytic and mucinous cells, viscous fluid
7. MCN	No connection to ductal system, females, ovarian-type stroma on histopathology, lacks squamous cells, thick background mucin with oncotic cells and histiocytes, neoplastic glandular epithelium, CEA elevated, amylase low.

Fig. 12. SCOPD. (*A*) Cytospin showing papillary-like cluster of squamous cells (Papanicolaou stain, ×400 magnification). (*B*) Cellblock showing a group of benign squamous cells with a luminal border of columnar cells (hematoxylin-eosin, ×400 magnification). (*C*) Mucicarmine stain demonstrating cytoplasmic mucin in the columnar cells (×400 magnification).

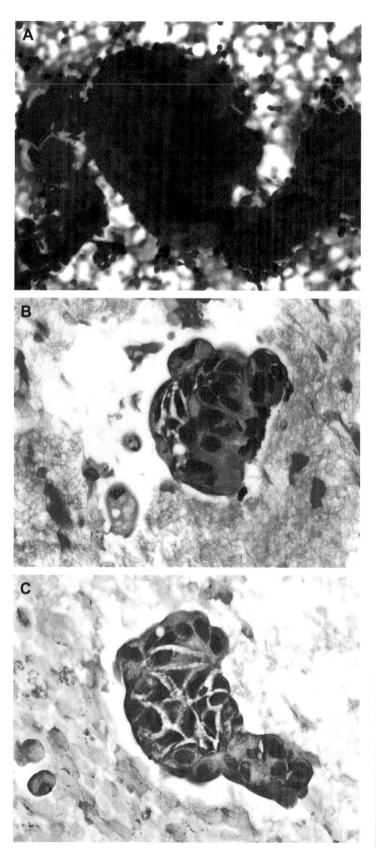

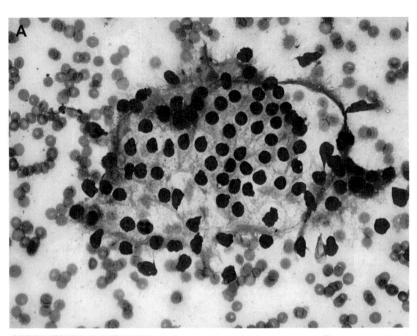

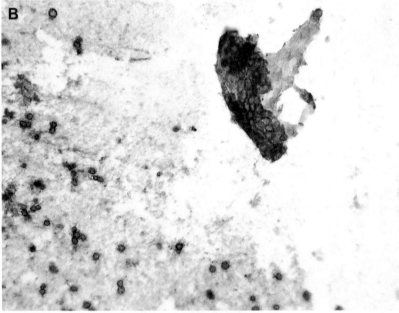

Fig. 13. SCA. (*A*) Monolayered sheet of neoplastic cells with clear cytoplasm, and round nuclei (Diff-Quik ×400 magnification). (*B*) IHC for GLUT1 performed on a smear of SCA (×400 magnification).

cystic neoplasms[65] and may be useful when this diagnosis is suspected and the sample is sufficiently cellular (see **Fig. 13**). GLUT1 is also expressed in PDAs with a clear cell pattern and high-grade dysplastic lesions. *KRAS* and *GNAS* mutations are negative in SCAs, and amylase and CEA cyst fluid levels are both low. Mutations in the *vHL* gene have been identified in a subset of SCAs.[66]

Neoplastic Mucinous Cysts: Mucinous Cystic Neoplasm and Intraductal Papillary Mucinous Neoplasm

Both MCN and IPMN are NMCs characterized by the proliferation of neoplastic mucinous, columnar epithelium lining cysts, or ducts. Both may progress to invasive pancreatic ductal carcinoma. MCN occurs exclusively in women, is not connected to the ductal system, is often located in the distal pancreas, shows ovarian-type stroma on histopathology, and has no risk of recurrence with complete resection as long as it is noninvasive. IPMN develops within the pancreatic ductal system and by definition connects with the ductal system. It occurs in both males and females and in all portions of the pancreas and does not have associated ovarian-type stroma. Because IPMN is usually multifocal, patients are at risk of recurrence after partial pancreatic resection and thus need to be carefully followed. The lining of both MCN and IPMN shows varying grades of dysplasia ranging from low grade to high grade.

In addition, the epithelial lining of IPMN is characterized into 4 subtypes: intestinal, pancreatobiliary, foveolar, and oncocytic. The oncocytic subtype has been reported as a separate entity, IOPN.[67] IPMN subtypes have characteristic histomorphology and IHC profile, with positive staining for MUC2 and CDX2 in intestinal type, MUC1 in pancreatobiliary type, MUC5AC in foveolar type, and MUC6 in oncocytic type IPMN.

Key Points
SEROUS CYSTADENOMA

1. Scant, nonviscous fluid.

2. Paucicellular to acellular aspirates.

3. Cuboidal cells with clear cytoplasm and round to oval nuclei, arranged in a monolayer, sometimes with fibrovascular stroma and stripped nuclei.

4. Low CEA and amylase.

5. PAS stains demonstrate cytoplasmic glycogen.

6. Expresses GLUT1.

7. Lacks *KRAS* and *GNAS* mutations.

8. Associated with mutations in *vHL* gene.

Serous cystadenoma	
Versus Differential Entity	**Distinguishing Feature(s) that Differ from Major Entity Under Discussion**
1. Gastric epithelium	Honeycomb morphology, thinner mucin, no oncotic cells, low CEA, absence of *KRAS* and *GNAS* mutations, contains mucins but not glycogen, GLUT1−, MUC5AC+
2. Small intestinal epithelium	Honeycomb morphology, goblet cells, lymphocytes, low CEA, absence of *KRAS* and *GNAS* mutations, absence of *vHL* mutation, lacks glycogen, GLUT1−, MUC2, and CDX2+
3. Benign ductal epithelium	Flat, uniform sheets, dense cytoplasm, glycogen−, GLUT1−, MUC1+
4. MCN	Mucinous epithelium and background mucin, CEA elevated, amylase low, *KRAS* mutations may be present, GLUT1−
5. IPMN	Connects to ductal system, same cytomorphology, viscous fluid, elevated CEA, *KRAS* and *GNAS* mutations may be present
6. IOPN	Connects to ductal system, same background, oncocytic and mucinous cells, viscous fluid, KRAS and GNAS mutations typically absent

The cytology of NMCs is characterized by background mucin and neoplastic mucin-containing epithelium. Aspiration may be difficult because the fluid is often extremely viscous. Gross examination shows highly viscous fluid that may be expressed from the needle as a mucin plug or as clear fluid with strands of mucus. The background mucin is usually thick and colloid-like with a pink hue on Papanicolaou stain. It may also be clumped or show ferning. Psammomatous calcifications may be seen in the mucin, along with degenerated oncotic cells[68] and macrophages (Fig. 14). The presence of thick background mucin with these characteristics indicates the presence of an NMC, even when neoplastic cells are not present. The cellularity of NMCs is variable. Cells may be singly dispersed or form sheets or papillary clusters or papillary tufts, and fibrovascular cores maybe seen in some examples. The sheets or clusters are subtly hypercellular and crowded, with cytoplasm that varies from columnar, with abundant mucin (Fig. 15A), to more rounded, with subtle vacuolization. Nuclei show variable atypia, the subtlest form being mild nuclear enlargement and hypochromasia with subtle nuclear membrane foldings. The hypochromatic nuclei may have small, peripheral nucleoli, similar to those seen in papillary thyroid carcinoma. Nuclear grooves and pseudoinclusions are also a feature (see Fig. 15B). Cytologic distinction between the intestinal, foveolar, and pancreatobiliary subtypes has not been reported. Alternatively, the oncocytic variant, IOPN, may be recognized on cytology, and the smear background also shows mucin. Abundant oncocytic cells, however, are seen interspersed with mucinous cells and fibrovascular cores are more prominent (Fig. 16).

Once a cyst is identified as cytologically compatible with an NMC, the next step is to assess the degree of dysplasia. The simplest approach is to assess for high-grade dysplasia and to report its presence or absence. High-grade epithelia atypia incorporates both high-grade dysplasia and invasive carcinoma. Features of high-grade epithelial atypia include an increased nuclear to cytoplasmic ratio, nuclear membrane irregularity, and abnormal chromatin distribution. Single dysplastic cells, which are small cells with high nuclear to cytoplasmic ratio and nuclear convolutions, are characteristic (Fig. 17).

Assessment of KRAS mutations by epithelial lining morphologic subtype in IPMN showed that 76% of gastric, 44% of intestinal, and 50% of the pancreatobiliary types harbored KRAS mutations. KRAS mutations have not

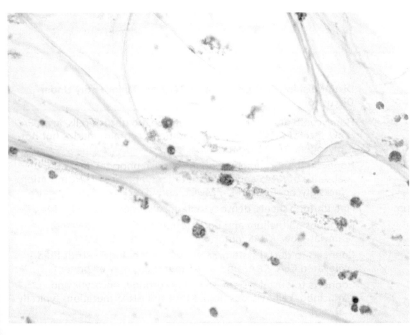

Fig. 14. Neoplastic mucinous cyst. Thick, pink background mucin with oncotic cells and histiocytes (Papanicolaou stain, ×400 magnification).

Fig. 15. NMC. (*A*) Nuclei with crowding, grooves and inclusions, and angulated nuclear shapes (hematoxylin-eosin, ×600 magnification). (*B*) Neoplastic cells with abundant, cytoplasmic mucin, and angulated nuclei with nuclear grooves (Papanicolaou stain, ×600 magnification).

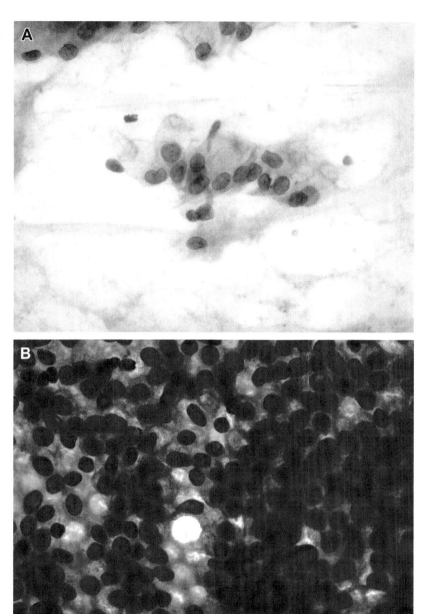

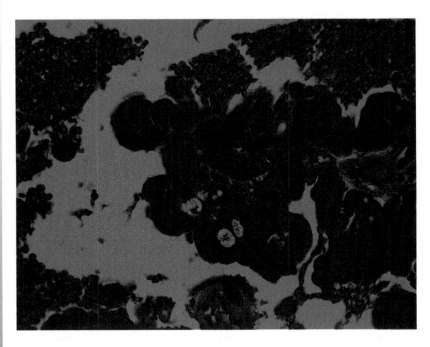

Fig. 16. Intraductal onco-cytic papillary neoplasm. Papillary cluster with cells with abundant, oncocytic cytoplasm, and mucin-containing cells (cellblock, hematoxylin-eosin, ×400 magnification).

been reported in the oncocytic neoplasms.[69] GNAS mutations were identified in 100% of the intestinal subtype, 51% of the gastric subtype, 71% of the pancreatobiliary subtype, and 0% of the oncocytic subtype.[70] The GNAS and KRAS mutations are not specific for grade of dysplasia or presence of invasive cancer.[70]

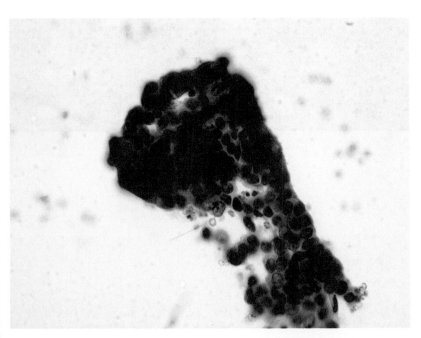

Fig. 17. NMC. The cells in this sheet show a high nu-clear to cytoplasmic ratio and nuclear membrane ab-normalities and abnormal-ities of the chromatin (Papanicolaou stain, ×400 magnification).

Key Points
INTRADUCTAL PAPILLARY MUCINOUS NEOPLASM

1. Intraductal and multifocal process.

2. No ovarian-type stroma on histopathology.

3. Viscous, mucinous fluid.

4. Cytology sample shows thick background mucin with oncotic cells and histiocytes.

5. Neoplastic glandular cells with variable cytoplasmic mucin and nuclear atypia.

6. Elevated CEA and amylase.

7. *KRAS* mutations in pancreatobiliary, foveolar and intestinal subtypes.

8. *GNAS* mutations.

Key Points
MUCINOUS CYSTIC NEOPLASM

1. Unifocal process.

2. Ovarian-type stroma on histopathology, no connection to ductal system.

3. Viscous, mucinous fluid.

4. Cytology sample shows thick background mucin with oncotic cells and histiocytes.

5. Neoplastic glandular cells with variable cytoplasmic mucin and nuclear atypia.

6. Elevated CEA and low amylase.

7. *KRAS* mutations.

8. Lacks *GNAS* mutations.

Intraductal papillary mucinous neoplasm

Versus Differential Entity	Distinguishing Feature(s) that Differ from Major Entity Under Discussion
1. Gastric epithelium	Honeycomb morphology, thinner mucin, no oncotic cells, low CEA, absence of *KRAS* and *GNAS* mutations
2. Small intestinal epithelium	Honeycomb morphology, goblet cells, lymphocytes, low CEA, absence of *KRAS* and *GNAS* mutations
3. SCOPD	Benign squamous epithelium with a single layer of columnar mucinous epithelium, dense background mucin, CEA and amylase elevated, lacks *KRAS* and *GNAS* mutations
4. Retention cyst	Histiocytes, background mucin, may have ductal epithelium, CEA elevated, lacks *KRAS* mutations and *GNAS* mutations
5. MCN	Does not connect with the ducts, same cytomorphology as IPMN, viscous fluid, elevated CEA, low amylase, *KRAS* mutations variably present, lacks *GNAS* mutations

Mucinous cystic neoplasm

Versus Differential Entity	Distinguishing Feature(s) that Differ from Major Entity Under Discussion
1. Gastric epithelium	Honeycomb morphology, thinner mucin, no oncotic cells, low CEA, absence of *KRAS* and *GNAS* mutations
2. Small intestinal epithelium	Honeycomb morphology, goblet cells, lymphocytes, low CEA, absence of *KRAS* and *GNAS* mutations
3. SCOPD	Benign squamous epithelium with a single layer of columnar mucinous epithelium, dense background mucin, CEA and amylase elevated, lacks *KRAS* and *GNAS* mutations
4. Retention cyst	Histiocytes, background mucin, may have ductal epithelium, CEA elevated, lacks *KRAS* mutations and *GNAS* mutations
5. IPMN	Connects to ductal system, same cytomorphology, viscous fluid, elevated CEA and amylase, *KRAS* and *GNAS* mutations may be present
6. IOPN	Connects to ductal system, same background, oncocytic and mucinous cells, viscous fluid

Invasive Carcinoma Arising from Intraductal Papillary Mucinous Neoplasm and Intraductal Oncocytic Papillary Neoplasm

There are different progression pathways for invasive adenocarcinoma developing from IPMN. Intestinal-type IPMN progresses to invasion with mucinous carcinoma, and all mucinous noncystic carcinomas are thought to arise from intestinal-type IPMN.[71] These are MUC2 and CDX2 positive. Pancreatobiliary and foveolar IPMNs progress to tubular carcinomas, whereas oncocytic IPMNs progress to invasive oncocytic carcinoma. The pancreatobiliary carcinomas are MUC1 positive. Oncocytic carcinomas express MUC6.

Invasion typically cannot be determined from only cyst fluid evaluation. Aspiration of a solid mural nodule in a mucinous cyst may prove diagnostic of invasion.[72] Coagulative necrosis or marked acute inflammation in aspirated material are concerning for invasion in an NMC.[73]

ROLE OF CYTOLOGY IN THE MANAGEMENT OF MUCINOUS CYSTS

Current management strategies are to resect all mucinous cysts that seem to be MCNs based on correlation with imaging findings. A mucinous cyst is suspected of being an IPMN if it connects to the ductal system or if the disease is multicentric. Preoperative assessment of patients with suspected IPMN now focuses on identifying patients who are at high risk of harboring high-grade dysplasia or invasive carcinoma using a combination of clinical history, gender, imaging characteristics, cytology, and cyst fluid biochemical and mutational analysis. The 2012 international consensus guidelines have identified certain features as high-risk stigmata for the presence of malignancy and other features as worrisome for malignancy. If worrisome features are present, patients are referred for EUS assessment with FNAB.[74] It is at this juncture that cytology becomes critical, because patients are referred for surgery if an aspirate is suspicious or positive for malignancy. The cytologic features that are predictive of high-grade dysplasia or adenocarcinoma have been grouped together as "high-grade epithelial atypia" because outright features of malignancy are infrequently present, and there is some overlap in the features of high-grade dysplasia with moderate dysplasia. The specific cytologic features that warrant classifying a cyst as showing high-grade dysplasia are discussed previously (see description of cytology for NMCs). At this time, there are no commercially available or validated tests that reliably identify cysts with high-grade dysplasia or invasive carcinoma.

Solid Neoplasms with Cystic Degeneration

PanNETs and SPNs are the two classic solid neoplasms that may undergo cystic degeneration and present as cystic or mixed solid and cystic masses on imaging studies. The cytomorphologic and ancillary studies are discussed previously (see discussion of solid neoplasms).

Rare Pancreatic and Extrapancreatic Cysts and Neoplasms

Peripancreatic and/or retroperitoneal cysts and cystic neoplasms that seem to be pancreatic in origin on radiologic studies comprised approximately 21% of percutaneously aspirated lesions.[75] Examples of non-neoplastic lesions include hydroureter, adrenal cyst, and mesothelial cyst. These lesions present a pitfall because they may be misdiagnosed as a primary pancreatic cyst.[75–77] These rare cysts or extrapancreatic lesions should be suspected if the imaging, clinical, cytologic, and cyst fluid ancillary studies do not correlate. Amylase measurements differentiate intrapancreatic from extrapancreatic cysts. Extrapancreatic cysts maintain amylase levels lower than serum levels.[45]

PRACTICAL APPLICATIONS

SOLID MASSES

Primary neoplasms of the pancreas presenting as solid masses have predominantly two distinct morphologic patterns. These are the solid stroma-rich ductal-type neoplasms, which are primarily PDAs, and the solid stroma-poor cellular neoplasms, which include neuroendocrine tumor, acinar cell carcinoma, SPN, and pancreatoblastoma. **Fig. 18** demonstrates an algorithmic approach incorporating morphology and ancillary studies into the differential diagnosis of solid lesions. A common pitfall in assessing solid neoplasms is misdiagnosis of acinar cell carcinoma, because this neoplasm may mimic neuroendocrine neoplasms on cytology. Therefore, when an acinar cell neoplasm is suspected, both acinar and neuroendocrine markers (trypsin, chymotrypsin, synaptophysin, and chromogranin A) should be routinely performed in tandem to ensure accurate diagnosis. Another potential pitfall is the combined acinar-neuroendocrine carcinoma, because this neoplasm may diffusely express synaptophysin. PanNET does not express CD10; therefore, if it expresses synaptophysin and CD10, it may represent a combined acinar-neuroendocrine carcinoma and should be worked up accordingly.

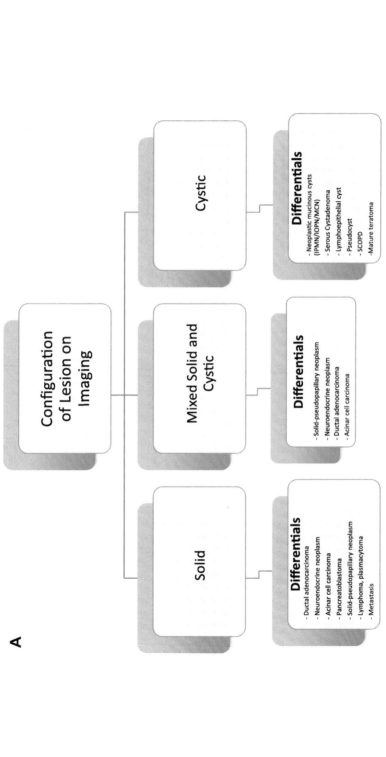

Fig. 18. Algorithms depicting approach to solid masses incorporating ancillary studies. (A) Algorithm 1—differential diagnosis of the most common solid and cystic pancreatic lesions encountered on imaging.

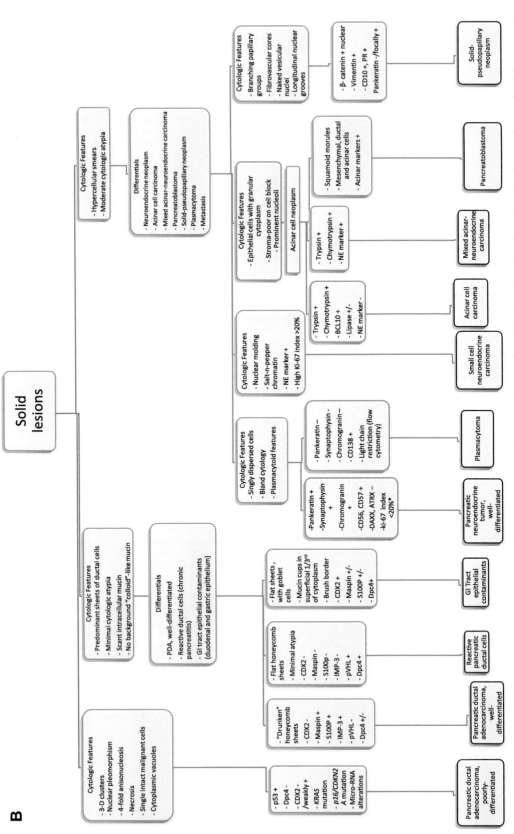

Fig. 18. (*continued*) Algorithms depicting approach to solid masses incorporating ancillary studies. (*B*) Algorithm 2—algorithm for the work-up of solid pancreatic lesions. (*, typically ki-67 index in <20% in well-differentiated PanNETs but exceptions do occur).

CYSTIC MASSES

Currently, work-up of cyst fluids is focused on distinguishing NMCs (IPMN/MCN) from nonmucinous cysts and neoplasms. Analysis of cyst fluid for cytology and ancillary studies are accurate at classifying pancreatic cysts as mucinous or nonmucinous.[78–80] The features of NMCs include thick, viscous fluid; elevated viscosity; characteristic background mucin; elevated CEA; KRAS mutations; and characteristic neoplastic epithelium. A diagnostic panel, including measurement of viscosity, cyst fluid CEA and amylase levels, cytology, and KRAS mutational analysis, is currently the most useful for this process. Although GNAS mutations have been identified in IPMN, assessment of these mutations currently is not routine.

GIT epithelial contaminants are present in all aspirates obtained by EUS-FNA and are a significant pitfall in the cytologic interpretation. Duodenal epithelium consists of enterocytes with interspersed goblet cells and is positive for MUC2 and CDX2. Gastric foveolar epithelium consists of tall columnar, mucin-containing cells that is MUC5AC positive. Duodenal epithelium is usually easy to recognize. Intestinal-type IPMN has the same immunophenotype, but when diagnostic cells are present, is typically recognizable as a neoplasm cytologically. Occasionally, however, duodenal epithelium may appear as atypical cell clusters, particularly on a cellblock. IHC for MUC1 may be beneficial in assessing an aspirate from the head of the pancreas, because it could differentiate pancreatobiliary epithelium from duodenal contaminant with atypical features. Foveolar epithelium is the most difficult, because it resembles low-grade IPMN, foveolar type. If a specimen consists of gastric contaminant only, the fluid is watery and nonviscous, has a low CEA level, and lacks KRAS and GNAS mutations. If the fluid does show features of an NMC, it is not necessary to differentiate foveolar contaminant from IPMN, foveolar type. The role of cytology in this specific situation is to identify cells with high-grade dysplasia. Adenocarcinoma with cystic degeneration may be identified if there is abundant, coagulative necrosis and overtly malignant-appearing cells. An algorithm illustrating a diagnostic approach to work-up of cystic lesions, incorporating cytology and ancillary studies, is depicted in **Fig. 19**.

PROGNOSTIC AND THERAPEUTIC APPLICATIONS OF ANCILLARY STUDIES IN SOLID AND CYSTIC PANCREATIC NEOPLASMS

The 3-tiered grading system for pancreatic neuroendocrine neoplasms has been shown to correlate strongly with outcome.[18,19] Such grading is only possible by counting mitoses or assessing a tumor's ki-67 proliferative index. Whether ki-67 indices should be performed on cytologic samples from pancreatic neuroendocrine neoplasms remains controversial. These tumors are notoriously heterogeneous and show marked variability in intratumoral mitotic activity. Additionally, cytologic samples are relatively hypocellular and often lack the 500 to 2000 tumor cells required for grading. Nonetheless, in cases where a cytologic sample is the only one available for evaluation, grading should be attempted by manually counting ki-67–positive tumor cells/500 tumor cells or by automated imaging (digital image analysis), both of which give comparable results on resections.[81] Manual counting and automated cellular imaging have been performed on cytologic samples for the grading of PanNETs and have shown comparable results in (a limited number of) corresponding resections.[2] In addition, the staining of pancreatic neuroendocrine tumors with CK19 is an independent prognostic marker and predictor of poor outcome and aggressive behavior.[82,83] Some investigators suggest that CK19 should routinely be performed on all pancreatic neuroendocrine tumors.[82]

Cytology is the only test in cyst fluids that provides a prognostic and therapeutic role, in that it is currently the only test that can identify IPMN with high-risk features (ie, high-grade dysplasia or adenocarcinoma). There are currently no ancillary studies with prognostic applications for cystic neoplasms.

Approximately 15% of PanNETs show somatic mutations of the mammalian target of rapamycin (mTOR) cell signaling pathway genes.[26] Alterations in the mTOR pathway have been exploited as therapeutic targets since the recent discovery of drugs directed specifically against this pathway.[84] BCL2 overexpression by PDNECs of pancreas can potentially be exploited with BCL2 antagonists in a manner similar to their hir current use in small cell carcinoma of lung which also overexpresses BCL2.[27]

There currently are no therapeutic applications of ancillary studies in cystic pancreatic neoplasms.

FUTURE TRENDS

WHOLE-EXOME SEQUENCING

Whole-exome sequencing of DNA extracted from the neoplastic epithelium of 8 IPMNs, 8 MCNs, 8 SPNs, and 8 SCAs identified recurrent mutations in components of ubiquitin dependent pathways.[66] Four of 8 SCAs harbored mutations

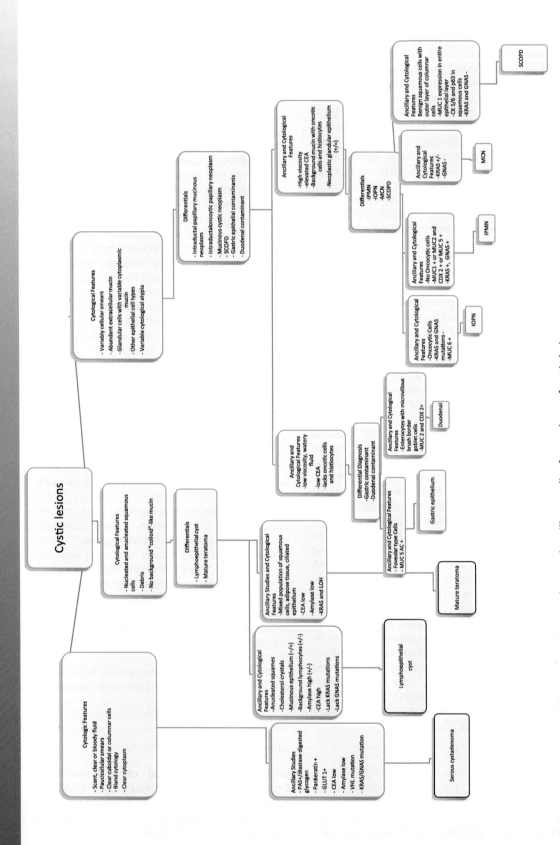

Fig. 19. Diagnostic algorithm incorporating cytology and ancillary studies for work-up of cystic lesions.

in *VHL* gene; 6 of 8 IPMNs, and 3 of 8 MCNs harbored mutations in *RNF43*, and all SPNs harbored mutations in *CTNNB1*. This suggests that a panel including mutational analysis of *VHL*, *RNF43*, and *CTNNB1* in addition to *KRAS* and *GNAS* could differentiate between SCA, IPMN, MCN, and SPN. Additional whole-exome sequencing studies may identify genes that are involved in the progression of IPMN and MCN to invasive cancer.

Whole-exome sequencing in PDA has demonstrated somatic mutations in *KRAS*, *p16/CDKN2A*, *DPC4/SMAD4*, and *TP53*. In the future, molecular studies can potentially be performed on aspirated material from solid neoplasms to identify these mutations and support a diagnosis of PDA.

miRNA SEQUENCING

In one study, miR-21, miR221, and miR17-3p showed significantly higher expression in the mucinous versus nonmucinous cysts (*P*<.01).[85] In another study, a subset of 18 miRNAs separated high-grade IPMN from low-grade IPMN, SCA, and uncommon cysts. A logistic regression model using 9 miRNAs allowed prediction of cyst pathology according to the need for resection (high-grade IPMN, PanNET, and SPN) versus conservative management (low-grade IPMN and SCA).[86] Another study identified 15 miRNAs that were differentially expressed between IPMN with low-grade or moderate dysplasia and IPMN with high-grade dysplasia or invasive carcinoma.[87] These studies suggest that miRNA profiling in pancreatic cyst fluids may prove useful for risk stratification in IPMN.

miRNA sequencing of PDA has revealed several miRNA alterations, some of which were identified on cellblock sections. In the future these studies can be performed on aspirated material and formalin-fixed paraffin embedded tissues to facilitate the diagnosis of PDA.

PROTEOMICS

Proteomic analysis is particularly applicable to pancreatic cyst fluids. One study identified homologs of amylase, solubilized molecules of 4 mucins, 4 solubilized CEA-related cell adhesion molecules, and 4 S100 homologs as candidate biomarkers to facilitate future pancreatic cyst diagnosis and risk-stratification.[88] Another study identified olfactomedin-4 and mucin-18 as markers of IPMN/MCN.[89] This technology could provide useful information in the future.

REFERENCES

1. Liu H, Shi J, Anandan V, et al. Reevaluation and identification of the best immunohistochemical panel (pVHL, Maspin, S100P, IMP-3) for ductal adenocarcinoma of the pancreas. Arch Pathol Lab Med 2012;136(6):601–9.
2. Fung A, Cohen C, Kavuri S, et al. Phosphohistone H3 and Ki-67 labeling indices in cytologic specimens from well differentiated neuroendocrine tumors of the gastrointestinal tract and pancreas: a comparative analysis using automated image cytometry. Acta Cytol 2013;57(5):501–8.
3. La Rosa S, Adsay V, Albarello L, et al. Clinicopathologic study of 62 acinar cell carcinomas of the pancreas: insights into the morphology and immunophenotype and search for prognostic markers. Am J Surg Pathol 2012;36(12):1782–95.
4. Ali S, Saleh H, Sethi S, et al. MicroRNA profiling of diagnostic needle aspirates from patients with pancreatic cancer. Br J Cancer 2012;107(8):1354–60.
5. Szafranska AE, Davison TS, John J, et al. MicroRNA expression alterations are linked to tumorigenesis and non-neoplastic processes in pancreatic ductal adenocarcinoma. Oncogene 2007;26(30):4442–52.
6. Jiao Y, Shi C, Edil BH, et al. DAXX/ATRX, MEN1, and mTOR pathway genes are frequently altered in pancreatic neuroendocrine tumors. Science 2011;331(6021):1199–203.
7. Alomari A, Eltoum I, Ustun B, et al. Endoscopic ultrasound guided fine needle aspiration (EUS-FNA) diagnosis of secondary tumors involving the pancreas: review of 102 cases. J Amer Society Cytopathol 2012;1(1S):S100 (Abstract).
8. Dodd LG, Evans DB, Symmans F, et al. Fine-needle aspiration of pancreatic extramedullary plasmacytoma: possible confusion with islet cell tumor. Diagn Cytopathol 1994;10(4):371–4 [discussion: 374–5].
9. Pitman MB, Deshpande V. Endoscopic ultrasound-guided fine needle aspiration cytology of the pancreas: a morphological and multimodal approach to the diagnosis of solid and cystic mass lesions. Cytopathology 2007;18(6):331–47.
10. Mitsuhashi T, Ghafari S, Chang CY, et al. Endoscopic ultrasound-guided fine needle aspiration of the pancreas: cytomorphological evaluation with emphasis on adequacy assessment, diagnostic criteria and contamination from the gastrointestinal tract. Cytopathology 2006;17(1):34–41.
11. Wood L, Adsay N, Hruban R. Molecular pathology of pancreatic cancer. In: Cheng L, Eble J, editors. Molecular surgical pathology. New York: Springer; 2013. p. 17–42.
12. Shen J, Cibas ES, Qian X. The immunohistochemicl expression pattern of SMAD4, p53 and CDX-2 is helpful in diagnosing pancreatic adenocarcinoma

in endoscopic ultrasound-guided fine needle aspiration (EUS-FNA). Mod Pathol 2007;20(Suppl 2):83A.

13. van Heek T, Rader AE, Offerhaus GJ, et al. K-ras, p53, and DPC4 (MAD4) alterations in fine-needle aspirates of the pancreas: a molecular panel correlates with and supplements cytologic diagnosis. Am J Clin Pathol 2002;117(5):755–65.

14. Scarpa A, Capelli P, Mukai K, et al. Pancreatic adenocarcinomas frequently show p53 gene mutations. Am J Pathol 1993;142(5):1534–43.

15. Wood LD, Hruban RH. Pathology and molecular genetics of pancreatic neoplasms. Cancer J 2012;18(6):492–501.

16. Jones S, Zhang X, Parsons D, et al. Core signaling pathways in human pancreatic cancers revealed by global genomic analyses. Science 2008;321(5897):1801.

17. Nagle JA, Wilbur DC, Pitman MB. Cytomorphology of gastric and duodenal epithelium and reactivity to B72.3: a baseline for comparison to pancreatic lesions aspirated by EUS-FNAB. Diagn Cytopathol 2005;33(6):381–6.

18. Klimstra DS, Modlin IR, Coppola D, et al. The pathologic classification of neuroendocrine tumors: a review of nomenclature, grading, and staging systems. Pancreas 2010;39(6):707–12.

19. Rindi G, Arnold R, Bosman F, et al. Nomenclature and classification of neuroendocrine tumors of the digestive system. In: Bosman F, Carneiro F, Hruban R, et al, editors. WHO classification of tumors of the digestive tract. Lyon (France): IARC Press; 2010. p. 322–6.

20. Chatzipantelis P, Salla C, Konstantinou P, et al. Endoscopic ultrasound-guided fine-needle aspiration cytology of pancreatic neuroendocrine tumors: a study of 48 cases. Cancer 2008;114(4):255–62.

21. Labate AM, Klimstra DL, Zakowski MF. Comparative cytologic features of pancreatic acinar cell carcinoma and islet cell tumor. Diagn Cytopathol 1997;16(2):112–6.

22. Jimenez-Heffernan JA, Vicandi B, Lopez-Ferrer P, et al. Fine needle aspiration cytology of endocrine neoplasms of the pancreas. Morphologic and immunocytochemical findings in 20 cases. Acta Cytol 2004;48(3):295–301.

23. Fung A, Cohen C, Kavuri S, et al. Interobserver variability in the quantification of MIB-1 labeling index on cytologic samples from well differentiated neuroendocrine tumors of the pancreas and gastrointestinal tract: a comparative analysis of three methods. Mod Pathol 2012;25(Suppl 2):512A.

24. Lin O, Olgac S, Green I, et al. Immunohistochemical staining of cytologic smears with MIB-1 helps distinguish low-grade from high-grade neuroendocrine neoplasms. Am J Clin Pathol 2003;120(2):209–16.

25. de Wilde RF, Heaphy CM, Maitra A, et al. Loss of ATRX or DAXX expression and concomitant acquisition of the alternative lengthening of telomeres phenotype are late events in a small subset of MEN-1 syndrome pancreatic neuroendocrine tumors. Mod Pathol 2012;25(7):1033–9.

26. Heaphy CM, de Wilde RF, Jiao Y, et al. Altered telomeres in tumors with ATRX and DAXX mutations. Science 2011;333(6041):425.

27. Small cell and large cell neuroendocrine carcinomas of the pancreas are genetically similar and distinct from well-differentiated pancreatic neuroendocrine tumors. Am J Surg Pathol 2012;36:173–84.

28. Stelow EB, Bardales RH, Shami VM, et al. Cytology of pancreatic acinar cell carcinoma. Diagn Cytopathol 2006;34(5):367–72.

29. Sigel CS, Klimstra DS. Cytomorphologic and immunophenotypical features of acinar cell neoplasms of the pancreas. Cancer Cytopathol 2013;121(8):459–70.

30. Ohike N, Kosmahl M, Kloppel G. Mixed acinar-endocrine carcinoma of the pancreas. A clinicopathological study and comparison with acinar-cell carcinoma. Virchows Arch 2004;445(3):231–5.

31. Pitman MB, Faquin WC. The fine-needle aspiration biopsy cytology of pancreatoblastoma. Diagn Cytopathol 2004;31(6):402–6.

32. Henke AC, Kelley CM, Jensen CS, et al. Fine-needle aspiration cytology of pancreatoblastoma. Diagn Cytopathol 2001;25(2):118–21.

33. Abraham SC, Wu TT, Hruban RH, et al. Genetic and immunohistochemical analysis of pancreatic acinar cell carcinoma: frequent allelic loss on chromosome 11p and alterations in the APC/beta-catenin pathway. Am J Pathol 2002;160(3):953–62.

34. Bardales RH, Centeno B, Mallery JS, et al. Endoscopic ultrasound-guided fine-needle aspiration cytology diagnosis of solid-pseudopapillary tumor of the pancreas: a rare neoplasm of elusive origin but characteristic cytomorphologic features. Am J Clin Pathol 2004;121(5):654–62.

35. Jani N, Dewitt J, Eloubeidi M, et al. Endoscopic ultrasound-guided fine-needle aspiration for diagnosis of solid pseudopapillary tumors of the pancreas: a multicenter experience. Endoscopy 2008;40(3):200–3.

36. Reid M. Cytology of the pancreas; A practical review for cytopathologists. In: Adsay N, Basturk O, editors. Current concepts in surgical pathology of the pancreas, vol. 4, 1st edition. Philadelphia: Saunders; 2011. p. 651–91.

37. Abraham SC, Klimstra DS, Wilentz RE, et al. Solid-pseudopapillary tumors of the pancreas are genetically distinct from pancreatic ductal adenocarcinomas and almost always harbor beta-catenin mutations. Am J Pathol 2002;160(4):1361–9.

38. Tanaka Y, Kato K, Notohara K, et al. Frequent beta-catenin mutation and cytoplasmic/nuclear accumulation in pancreatic solid-pseudopapillary neoplasm. Cancer Res 2001;61(23):8401–4.

39. Chetty R, Serra S. Membrane loss and aberrant nuclear localization of E-cadherin are consistent features of solid pseudopapillary tumour of the pancreas. An immunohistochemical study using two antibodies recognizing different domains of the E-cadherin molecule. Histopathology 2008; 52(3):325–30.

40. Zhu LC, Sidhu GS, Cassai ND, et al. Fine-needle aspiration cytology of pancreatoblastoma in a young woman: report of a case and review of the literature. Diagn Cytopathol 2005;33(4):258–62.

41. Nakatani Y, Masudo K, Nozawa A, et al. Biotin-rich, optically clear nuclei express estrogen receptor-beta: tumors with morules may develop under the influence of estrogen and aberrant beta-catenin expression. Hum Pathol 2004;35(7):869–74.

42. Adsay NV, Andea A, Basturk O, et al. Secondary tumors of the pancreas: an analysis of a surgical and autopsy database and review of the literature. Virchows Arch 2004;444(6):527–35.

43. Reid M, Sullivan H, Henderson-Jackson E, et al. Metastatic tumors of the pancreas diagnosed by fine needle aspiration: a multi-institutional analysis of 38 cases. Mod Pathol 2013;26(Suppl 2):100A.

44. Niess H, Conrad C, Kleespies A, et al. Surgery for metastasis to the pancreas: is it safe and effective? J Surg Oncol 2013;107(8):859–64.

45. Lewandrowski K, Lee J, Southern J, et al. Cyst fluid analysis in the differential diagnosis of pancreatic cysts: a new approach to the preoperative assessment of pancreatic cystic lesions. AJR Am J Roentgenol 1995;164(4):815–9.

46. Centeno BA, Stockwell JW, Lewandrowski KB. Cyst fluid cytology and chemical features in a case of lymphoepithelial cyst of the pancreas: a rare and difficult preoperative diagnosis. Diagn Cytopathol 1999;21(5):328–30.

47. Leung KK, Ross WA, Evans D, et al. Pancreatic cystic neoplasm: the role of cyst morphology, cyst fluid analysis, and expectant management. Ann Surg Oncol 2009;16(10):2818–24.

48. Brugge WR, Lewandrowski K, Lee-Lewandrowski E, et al. Diagnosis of pancreatic cystic neoplasms: a report of the cooperative pancreatic cyst study. Gastroenterology 2004;126(5):1330–6.

49. Pitman MB, Lewandrowski K, Shen J, et al. Pancreatic cysts: preoperative diagnosis and clinical management. Cancer Cytopathol 2010; 118(1):1–13.

50. Belsley NA, Pitman MB, Lauwers GY, et al. Serous cystadenoma of the pancreas: limitations and pitfalls of endoscopic ultrasound-guided fine-needle aspiration biopsy. Cancer 2008;114(2):102–10.

51. Khalid A, Zahid M, Finkelstein SD, et al. Pancreatic cyst fluid DNA analysis in evaluating pancreatic cysts: a report of the PANDA study. Gastrointest Endosc 2009;69(6):1095–102.

52. Panarelli NC, Sela R, Schreiner AM, et al. Commercial molecular panels are of limited utility in the classification of pancreatic cystic lesions. Am J Surg Pathol 2012;36(10):1434–43.

53. Nikiforova MN, Khalid A, Fasanella KE, et al. Integration of KRAS testing in the diagnosis of pancreatic cystic lesions: a clinical experience of 618 pancreatic cysts. Mod Pathol 2013;26(11): 1478–87.

54. Wu J, Matthaei H, Maitra A, et al. Recurrent GNAS mutations define an unexpected pathway for pancreatic cyst development. Sci Transl Med 2011; 3(92):92ra66.

55. Jorda M, Essenfeld H, Garcia E, et al. The value of fine-needle aspiration cytology in the diagnosis of inflammatory pancreatic masses. Diagn Cytopathol 1992;8(1):65–7.

56. Centeno BA, Lewandrowski KB, Warshaw AL, et al. Cyst fluid cytologic analysis in the differential diagnosis of pancreatic cystic lesions. Am J Clin Pathol 1994;101(4):483–7.

57. Gonzalez Obeso E, Murphy E, Brugge W, et al. Pseudocyst of the pancreas: the role of cytology and special stains for mucin. Cancer Cytopathol 2009;117(2):101–7.

58. Hughes JH, Cohen MB. Fine-needle aspiration of the pancreas. Pathology (Phila) 1996;4(2): 389–407.

59. Liu J, Shin HJ, Rubenchik I, et al. Cytologic features of lymphoepithelial cyst of the pancreas: two preoperatively diagnosed cases based on fine-needle aspiration. Diagn Cytopathol 1999;21(5): 346–50.

60. Mandavilli SR, Port J, Ali SZ. Lymphoepithelial cyst (LEC) of the pancreas: cytomorphology and differential diagnosis on fine-needle aspiration (FNA). Diagn Cytopathol 1999;20(6):371–4.

61. Policarpio-Nicolas ML, Shami VM, Kahaleh M, et al. Fine-needle aspiration cytology of pancreatic lymphoepithelial cysts. Cancer 2006; 108(6):501–6.

62. Raval JS, Zeh HJ, Moser AJ, et al. Pancreatic lymphoepithelial cysts express CEA and can contain mucous cells: potential pitfalls in the preoperative diagnosis. Mod Pathol 2010;23(11):1467–76.

63. Othman M, Basturk O, Groisman G, et al. Squamoid cyst of pancreatic ducts: a distinct type of cystic lesion in the pancreas. Am J Surg Pathol 2007;31(2):291–7.

64. Huang P, Staerkel G, Sneige N, et al. Fine-needle aspiration of pancreatic serous cystadenoma: cytologic features and diagnostic pitfalls. Cancer 2006; 108(4):239–49.

65. Basturk O, Singh R, Kaygusuz E, et al. GLUT-1 expression in pancreatic neoplasia: implications in pathogenesis, diagnosis, and prognosis. Pancreas 2011;40(2):187–92.

66. Wu J, Jiao Y, Dal Molin M, et al. Whole-exome sequencing of neoplastic cysts of the pancreas reveals recurrent mutations in components of ubiquitin-dependent pathways. Proc Natl Acad Sci U S A 2011;108(52):21188–93.

67. Adsay NV, Adair CF, Heffess CS, et al. Intraductal oncocytic papillary neoplasms of the pancreas. Am J Surg Pathol 1996;20(8):980–94.

68. Xiao GQ. Fine-needle aspiration of cystic pancreatic mucinous tumor: oncotic cell as an aiding diagnostic feature in paucicellular specimens. Diagn Cytopathol 2009;37(2):111–6.

69. Patel SA, Adams R, Goldstein M, et al. Genetic analysis of invasive carcinoma arising in intraductal oncocytic papillary neoplasm of the pancreas. Am J Surg Pathol 2002;26(8):1071–7.

70. Dal Molin M, Matthaei H, Wu J, et al. Clinicopathological correlates of activating GNAS mutations in intraductal papillary mucinous neoplasm (IPMN) of the pancreas. Ann Surg Oncol 2013;20(12):3802–8.

71. Adsay NV, Merati K, Basturk O, et al. Pathologically and biologically distinct types of epithelium in intraductal papillary mucinous neoplasms: delineation of an "intestinal" pathway of carcinogenesis in the pancreas. Am J Surg Pathol 2004;28(7):839–48.

72. Tomaszewska R, Popiela T, Karcz D, et al. Infiltrating carcinoma arising in intraductal papillary-mucinous tumor of the pancreas. Diagn Cytopathol 1998;18(6):445–8.

73. Michaels PJ, Brachtel EF, Bounds BC, et al. Intraductal papillary mucinous neoplasm of the pancreas: cytologic features predict histologic grade. Cancer 2006;108(3):163–73.

74. Tanaka M, Fernandez-del Castillo C, Adsay V, et al. International consensus guidelines 2012 for the management of IPMN and MCN of the pancreas. Pancreatology 2012;12(3):183–97.

75. Centeno BA, Warshaw AL, Mayo-Smith W, et al. Cytologic diagnosis of pancreatic cystic lesions. A prospective study of 28 percutaneous aspirates. Acta Cytol 1997;41(4):972–80.

76. Sperti C, Cappellazzo F, Pasquali C, et al. Cystic neoplasms of the pancreas: problems in differential diagnosis. Am Surg 1993;59(11):740–5.

77. Malhotra R, Evans R, Bhawan J, et al. A malignant gastric leiomyoblastoma presenting as an infected pseudocyst of the pancreas. Am J Gastroenterol 1988;83(4):452–6.

78. Cizginer S, Turner B, Bilge AR, et al. Cyst fluid carcinoembryonic antigen is an accurate diagnostic marker of pancreatic mucinous cysts. Pancreas 2011;40(7):1024–8.

79. Yoshizawa K, Nagai H, Sakurai S, et al. Clonality and K-ras mutation analyses of epithelia in intraductal papillary mucinous tumor and mucinous cystic tumor of the pancreas. Virchows Arch 2002;441(5):437–43.

80. Khalid A, Finkelstein S, McGrath K. Molecular diagnosis of solid and cystic lesions of the pancreas. Gastroenterol Clin North Am 2004;33(4):891–906.

81. Tang LH, Gonen M, Hedvat C, et al. Objective quantification of the Ki67 proliferative index in neuroendocrine tumors of the gastroenteropancreatic system: a comparison of digital image analysis with manual methods. Am J Surg Pathol 2012;36(12):1761–70.

82. Jain R, Fischer S, Serra S, et al. The use of Cytokeratin 19 (CK19) immunohistochemistry in lesions of the pancreas, gastrointestinal tract, and liver. Appl Immunohistochem Mol Morphol 2010;18(1):9–15.

83. Deshpande V, Muzikansky A, Fernandez del Castillo C. Cytokeratin 19 is a powerful predictor of survival in pancreatic endocrine tumors. Mod Pathol 2003;16(Suppl):272A.

84. Yao JC, Shah MH, Ito T, et al. Everolimus for advanced pancreatic neuroendocrine tumors. N Engl J Med 2011;364(6):514–23.

85. Ryu JK, Matthaei H, Dal Molin M, et al. Elevated microRNA miR-21 levels in pancreatic cyst fluid are predictive of mucinous precursor lesions of ductal adenocarcinoma. Pancreatology 2011;11(3):343–50.

86. Matthaei H, Wylie D, Lloyd MB, et al. miRNA biomarkers in cyst fluid augment the diagnosis and management of pancreatic cysts. Clin Cancer Res 2012;18(17):4713–24.

87. Lubezky N, Loewenstein S, Ben-Haim M, et al. MicroRNA expression signatures in intraductal papillary mucinous neoplasm of the pancreas. Surgery 2013;153(5):663–72.

88. Ke E, Patel BB, Liu T, et al. Proteomic analyses of pancreatic cyst fluids. Pancreas 2009;38(2):e33–42.

89. Cuoghi A, Farina A, Z'Graggen K, et al. Role of proteomics to differentiate between benign and potentially malignant pancreatic cysts. J Proteome Res 2011;10(5):2664–70.

Ancillary Studies, Including Immunohistochemistry and Molecular Studies, in Lung Cytology

Fernando Schmitt, MD, PhD, FIAC[a,b,]*, José Carlos Machado, PhD[b]

KEYWORDS

- Lung cytology • Immunohistochemistry • Molecular testing • EGFR • ALK

ABSTRACT

The importance of cytologic techniques for investigation of respiratory conditions has been recognized since the earliest days of clinical cytology. Cytology is able to detect most of mycoses and parasitic and viral infections based on the morphologic recognition of these agents. The most relevant application of lung cytology today is in the diagnosis and management of lung cancer; approximately 70% of those cancers are diagnosed at a late stage and are unresectable. This article addresses the most common ancillary techniques, such as special stains, immunocytochemistry, and molecular testing, used to refine the cytologic diagnosis of lung cancer and to guide personalized therapy.

OVERVIEW

The importance of cytologic techniques for investigation of respiratory conditions has been recognized since the earliest days of clinical cytology. The study of cellular specimens from the respiratory tract is established as a vital diagnostic procedure in the evaluation of patients with suspected lung inflammatory/infectious or neoplastic diseases. The study of sputum, bronchial washings, bronchial aspirates, bronchial brushings, bronchoalveolar lavage specimens, and fine-needle aspirates (FNAs) provides the morphologic basis for these diagnoses. Cytology is able to detect most of mycoses and parasitic and viral infections based on the morphologic recognition of these agents. The importance of the application of ancillary techniques in this field to detect some microorganisms, however, for example acid-fast special staining in tuberculosis,[1] has been recognized for a long time.

The most relevant application of lung cytology today is in the diagnosis and management of lung cancer because approximately 70% of those cancers are diagnosed at a late stage and are unresectable. Small biopsies and cytology are the primary material used for establishing diagnosis and for study of molecular markers that can drive therapy.[2–4] The identification of EGFR-positive adenocarcinomas (ADCs) permits the use of tyrosine kinase inhibitors (TKIs); and the recognition of squamous cell carcinoma (SqCC) avoids the use of bevacizumab, which has been linked to serious bleeding in this subset of lung cancer patients.[3–5] Moreover, ADC with ALK rearrangements is responsive to crizotinib,[3,6] and ADC or non–small

The authors have no relevant financial interest in the products or companies described in this article.

[a] Department of Laboratory Medicine & Pathobiology, Faculty of Medicine, University of Toronto, University Health Network Toronto General Hospital, 200 Elizabeth Street, 11E-215B Toronto, ON M5G 2C4, Canada; [b] IPATIMUP, Institute of Molecular Pathology and Immunology of Porto University, Rua Dr Roberto Frias S/N, 4200-465, Porto, Portugal

* Corresponding author. IPATIMUP, Institute of Molecular Pathology and Immunology of Porto University, Rua Dr Roberto Frias S/N, 4200-465, Porto, Portugal.

E-mail address: fernando.schmitt@ipatimup.pt

Surgical Pathology 7 (2014) 35–46
http://dx.doi.org/10.1016/j.path.2013.10.005

surgpath.theclinics.com

cell lung carcinoma (NSCLC), not otherwise specified (NSCLC-NOS), is more responsive than SqCC to pemetrexed.[7] This article addresses the most common ancillary techniques, such as special stains, immunocytochemistry (ICC), and molecular testing, used to refine the cytologic diagnosis of lung cancer as well as to guide personalized therapy for patients.

CYTOLOGIC DIFFERENTIAL DIAGNOSIS

The most common subtypes of lung cancer can be diagnosed on cytology if the established morphologic criteria are present.[2,3,8] Cytologically, ADCs are characterized by the presence of different architectural patterns, including cell balls, papillary fronds, and cohesive clusters with acinar structures, and the individual cells show delicate cytoplasm, varying in appearance from homogenous to extremely vacuolated. The nuclei are enlarged, with finely to coarsely granular chromatin, and show prominent and centrally placed nucleoli (Fig. 1). SqCC is recognized by three main morphologic characteristics: keratinization (easily recognized in Papanicolaou stain as orange or red cytoplasm), pearls, and intercellular bridges.

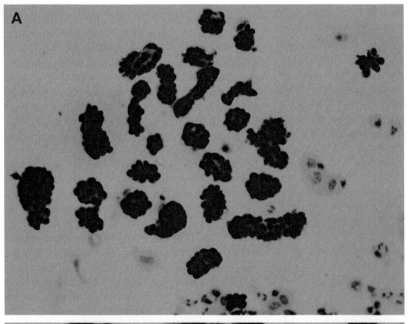

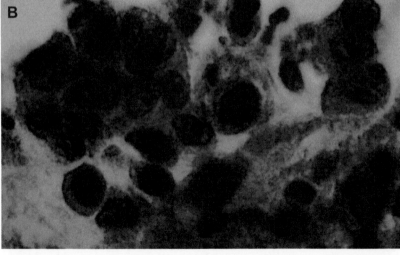

Fig. 1. ADC. (*A*) LBC preparation showing ADC cells with papillary configuration (Papanicolaou stain, original magnification ×20). (*B*) Neoplastic cells with large delicate cytoplasm and clearly malignant nuclei with prominent nucleoli (LBC preparation, Papanicolaou stain; original magnification ×60).

SqCC often present as geographic broad sheets of cells and show peripheral spindling. The cytoplasm is usually dense and homogeneous, and nuclei are hyperchromatic (**Fig. 2**). When ADCs and SqCCs are poorly differentiated, these morphologic criteria may not be as distinct, and ancillary studies, such as special stains and ICC, may be necessary to make a more-specific diagnosis. The presence of densely eosinophilic cytoplasm or sharp intercytoplasmic borders in the absence of frank keratinization, pearls, or intercellular bridges is insufficient for a definitive diagnosis of SqCC.

Small cell lung carcinoma (SCLC) has characteristic findings on cytology, including small cells arranged in loose clusters and single cells, nuclear molding, scant cytoplasm, nuclei with salt-and-pepper chromatin with no or small nucleoli, and frequent associated necrosis and mitosis. Large cell neuroendocrine carcinoma (LCNEC) is

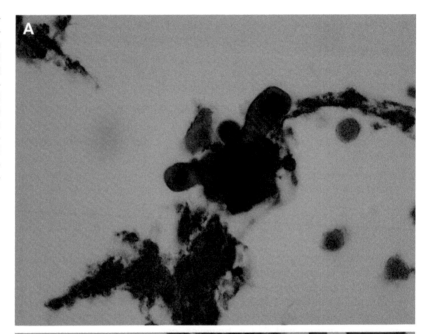

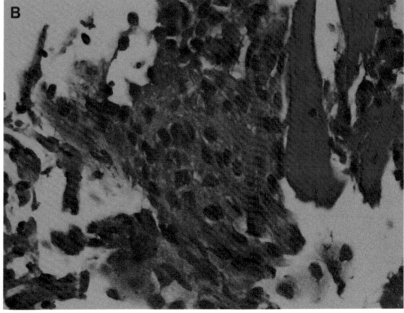

Fig. 2. SqCC. (*A*) Neoplastic cells showing keratinizing cytoplasm with hyperchromatic nuclei and necrotic background (LBC preparation, Papanicolaou stain; original magnification ×40). (*B*) Neoplastic cells with dense cytoplasm and intercellular bridges (cell block preparation, hematoxylin-eosin stain; original magnification ×40).

characterized by smears with intermediate to large pleomorphic single cells or groups with more abundant cytoplasm, prominent nucleoli, and a "dirty" background. These groups have peripheral palisading and not infrequently form rosette-like structures. Poorly differentiated ADCs, however, can share some of these characteristics; hence, neuroendocrine markers (CD56, chromogranin, and synaptophysin) are essential for differential diagnosis between these two entities. In this situation, SCLC and LCNEC, similar to ADC, can also stain positive with thyroid transcription factor (TTF)-1.[9]

Although histologic heterogeneity can occur in lung cancer, and small biopsy and/or cytology may not be representative of the total tumor, combined histologic types are rarely encountered and comprise less than 5% of all resected NSCLCs.[3] Also, it is not possible to diagnose ADC in situ, minimally invasive ADC, large cell carcinoma, or pleomorphic carcinoma from a small biopsy or cytology. The diagnosis of large cell carcinoma requires extensive sampling of the tumor to exclude a differentiated component. Therefore, if differentiation is not present, these cases should be classified as NSCLC-NOS. The diagnosis of pleomorphic carcinoma requires also a resection specimen with a component of at least 10%

spindle and/or giant cell component. Pleomorphic cells found in cytologic specimens with a component of ADC, SqCC, or even large cells should be noted in the cytology report (ie, NSCLC, favor ADC with giant and/or spindle cell features, with a comment noting that this could be a pleomorphic carcinoma).[3]

ANCILLARY STUDIES, DIAGNOSTIC

SPECIAL STAINS

The use of special stains in lung cytology is more related to the diagnosis of infections. Gram staining for bacteria, silver-based stains for fungi and *Pneumocystis jiroveci*, and acid-fast staining for mycobacteriosis, among other stains, are used. In lung cancer, mucin stains (diastase/periodic acid–Schiff, alcian blue, and mucicarmine) are applied to recognize ADCs. In clinical practice, however, for the most part, mucin stains have been replaced by ICC stains (Table 1).

IMMUNOCYTOCHEMISTRY

Cytology laboratories process different types of preparations, such as FNAs, cell suspensions,

Table 1
Common special stains used in lung cytology

Stain	Application
Ziehl-Neelsen (acid-fast bacillus)	Detect and identify acid-fast bacilli in tissue. Bacilli are rod-shaped bacterial organisms. A primary function of this stain is to identify tuberculosis
Modified Gomori methenamine silver stain	Observation of fungi and some opportunistic organisms, such as pneumocystis jiroveci.
Periodic–acid Schiff	Mainly used for staining structures containing a high proportion of carbohydrates, such as glycogen, glycoproteins, and proteoglycans typically found in connective tissues and in mucus and basement membranes. Often used to detect mucus in ADC and in cases of suspected fungal infections.
Alcian blue	Normally prepared at pH 2.5 and is used to identify acid mucopolysaccharides and acidic mucins. Excessive amounts of nonsulfated acidic mucosubstances are seen in mesotheliomas.
Mucicarmine	A valuable technique for the evaluation of acid mucins. In addition, it is useful for staining the capsule of the fungus *Cryptococcus neoformans*.

and various types of exfoliative collections. Proper specimen processing is of utmost importance for any ancillary technique. The most commonly used preparations are direct smears, Cytospin centrifugations, cell blocks, and liquid-based cytology (LBC) preparations.

Direct smears are prepared from FNA material, brushings, or sediment fresh effusions. After being air-dried, smears should be fixed in formalin followed by alcohol. Immunostaining usually performs well in nuclear antigens, such as TTF-1, P63, and P40, but is less suitable for membrane or cytoplasmic antigens because of high background staining secondary to cell damage caused by smearing. The cytomorphology of direct smears is excellent, but the number of slides is usually limited and prevents the use of an extensive marker panel. Although the cost of preparation of direct smears is low, the amount of antibodies needed to cover the entire slide is high.

Cytospin preparations are prepared from cell suspensions in nonfixative solutions, such as RPMI, FNA material, or effusions. Cytospin material offers an excellent source of staining for most antibodies although various fixatives have to be used. This technique, however, is less suitable for specimens with a rich admixture of blood or mucus. In most cases, many Cytospin slides can be prepared, which allows the use of a panel with many antibodies. LBC preparation systems are available in most cytology laboratories and can be stained with various antibodies to nuclear, cytoplasmic, and membrane-bound antigens in a reproducible way. Several slides can be produced from LBC material, which allows a complete immunologic work-up in most cases.

Cell blocks can be prepared from all types of cytologic specimens and perform in a highly reproducible fashion when stained with most antibodies. One distinct advantage of cell blocks is that many slides can be prepared for an extensive panel of immunostains. In addition, the quality control of cell block staining is identical to that of histopathology. This technique is time-consuming, but the cost is comparable to that of the Cytospin technique. Because most molecular techniques are now standardized for paraffin-embedded tissues, they can apply directly to cell block preparations with excellent results.

PRACTICAL APPLICATIONS OF IMMUNOCYTOCHEMISTRY

Often, cytology is the only material available for diagnosis in lung cancer; therefore, a panel of well-defined markers must be used to refine a diagnosis of NSCLC to ADC or SqCC. Several studies have demonstrated that, in general, ADC is positive for TTF-1, napsin A, and CK7, whereas most SqCCs express P40, P63, and/or CK5/6.[4,10] Because it is important not to exhaust the available diagnostic sample and ensure that enough material is available for an eventual molecular study, it is useful to validate a minimalist ICC panel. Pelosi and colleagues[11] provided evidence that a two-hit minimalist approach on cytologic material based on P40 and TTF-1 is helpful in the distinction between ADC and SqCC. The authors and colleagues showed that P40, a polyclonal antibody that recognizes one of the isoforms of P63 (DNP63) is more specific than the monoclonal P63 antibody (4A4) in recognizing SqCC (97% vs 69% of specificity).[12] Another possibility is the use of cocktails of nuclear and cytoplasmic markers (TTF-1/CK 5/6 or P63/napsin A) that can allow for utilization of fewer ICC studies yet multiple antibodies.[10,13]

TTF-1 and P40 are generally mutually exclusive[14]; therefore, if a case is positive for an ADC marker (ie, TTF-1 and/or mucin) and a negative for a squamous marker (ie, P40 or P63), it should be classified as NSCLC, favor ADC (Fig. 3). Cases positive for a squamous maker and a negative for an ADC marker should be classified as NSCLC, favor SqCC. Virtually all tumors that coexpress TTF-1 and P63 are ADCs and this coexpression has been reported in ALK-positive cases.[15] TTF-1 and P63 seen in different populations of tumor cells suggest the possibility of adenosquamous carcinoma.

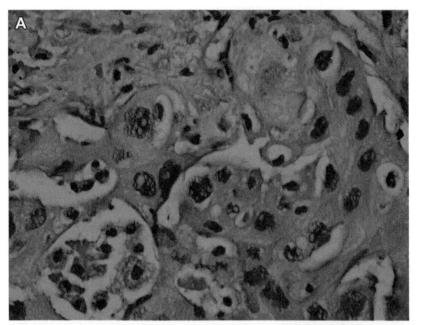

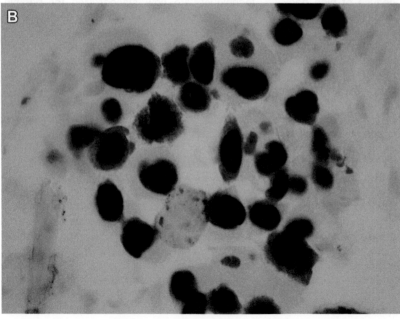

Fig. 3. NSCLC, favor ADC. (A) Solid tumor with no distinct squamous, acinar, papillary, or mucinous differentiation (cell block preparation, hematoxylin-eosin stain; original magnification ×40). (B) Tumor cells are strongly positive for TTF-1 (ICC for TTF-1, original magnification ×40).

Table 2
Common immunocytochemistry markers used in lung cytology

Lung Cancer Subtype	Markers					
	TTF-1	Napsin A	P63	P40	CK5/6	Neuroendocrine Markers
ADC	+/−[a]	+	−/+	−	−	−
SqCC	−	−	+	+	+	−
SCLC	+	−	−	−	−	+
NSCLC-NOS	+/−	−	−	−	−	−
Metastatic carcinoma	−/+	−	−/+	−/+	−/+	−/+

[a] Especially mucinous ADC.

ICC also has an important role in differentiating NSCLC from SCLC and LCNEC. In these cases, a panel of immunostains composed of TTF-1, CD56 NCAM, synaptophysin or chromogranin, CK5/6, and P63/P40 help differentiate SCLC from a small cell variant of SqCC.[9] There is a minority of cases where the diagnosis remains NSCLC-NOS, because no differentiation can be established by routine morphology and ICC (Table 2).[3]

If both TTF-1 and P40 are negative in a tumor that lacks definite squamous or glandular differentiation, performing a cytokeratin stain may be considered to confirm that the tumor is a carcinoma. If cytokeratin is negative, further stains may be needed to exclude other malignancies with epithelioid morphology, such as melanoma, lymphoma, and mesothelioma, among other malignancies. If cytomorphology of ADC is recognized but it is TTF-1 negative (primary lung ADCs can be TTF-1 negative in approximately 20%–30% of cases), additional markers, such as CDX2, CK20, estrogen receptor, progesterone receptor, and prostate-specific antigen, should be considered to exclude metastasis from other sites, such as gastrointestinal tract, breast, or prostate, in the appropriate clinical setting. Having said that, invasive mucinous ADCs or colloid lung ADCs are TTF-1 negative and can express CDX2. In these cases, clinical correlation is needed to exclude pancreas or colon metastasis.

Key Points
IMMUNOCYTOCHEMISTRY IN LUNG CYTOLOGY

1. All cytology preparations can be used to perform ICC; however, cell blocks are more reproducible, allow use of controls, and are standardized for molecular studies.

2. A minimalist panel of markers should be validated to preserve material for eventual molecular studies.

3. TTF-1 and P40 are mutually exclusive and are helpful in distinguishing ADC from SqCC.

4. P40 Is more specific than monoclonal P63 antibody in recognizing SqCC.

5. Napsin-A and CK5/6 can be used to distinguish ADC from SqCC, especially when used together in cocktails of nuclear and cytoplasmic markers.

6. Tumors that coexpress TTF-1 and P63 are usually ADCs, and this coexpression is associated with ALK-positive cases.

7. Mucinous lung ADCs are TTF-1 negative and can express CDX2.

8. TTF-1–negative nonmucinous ADC in the lung requires additional markers to exclude metastases.

9. Poorly differentiated tumors that are TTF-1 and P63 negative and lack squamous or glandular differentiation should be stained for cytokeratin to confirm epithelial differentiation.

MOLECULAR TESTING

In lung cytology, the major application of molecular testing is to study therapeutic targets rather than establish a diagnosis. It is critical to highlight that in addition to making a correct morphologic diagnosis, pathologists have a new responsibility: to manage these small biopsy and cytology samples strategically, so there is sufficient tissue preserved for molecular studies (ie, use the minimum specimen necessary for an accurate diagnosis to preserve as much tissue as possible for potential molecular studies).[3,16] This strategic approach (**Fig. 4**) should be multidisciplinary and begins with the method of retrieving tissue for diagnosis. Communication with other clinicians who participate in the diagnosis and management of lung cancer (radiologists, surgeons, oncologists, and pulmonologists) can aid in determining the best way to obtain adequate material not only for diagnosis but also for molecular testing. Onsite evaluation and assessment of biopsy adequacy in collaboration with the molecular laboratory are critical steps in selecting the best material for molecular testing. Exhausting substantial amounts of tissue or cells to establish a diagnosis of ADC or SqCC, such as multiple recuts/deepers and extensive panel of immunohistochemistry stains, may not provide an advantage over routine microscopy with a limited ICC work-up.[3]

THERAPEUTIC AND PROGNOSTIC APPLICATIONS

The most important molecular discoveries associated with lung cancer therapeutics are related to the use of selective TKIs targeting EGFR mutations and the ALK fusion genes. All ADCs must be tested routinely for the presence of *EGFR* mutation and, if negative, tested for the ALK translocations.[17] EGFR mutations in lung ADCs are mainly associated with female nonsmokers and are more often found in better differentiated ADCs with or without mucinous component. These patients benefit from EGFR-TKI therapy, and a first-line treatment with EGFR-TKI is now standard of care in these patients. In unselected advanced NSCLC patients, gefitinib and erlotinib produce response rates of 8% to 9%, with a median time to progression of approximately 3 months.[18] In contrast, advanced NSCLC patients selected on the basis of activating EGFR mutations in their tumors show response rates of 68%, with a mean progression-free survival and time to progression of approximately 12 months.[19–21]

Molecular detection of EGFR mutation is currently the most accurate method of selecting these patients.[17] A recent review of the literature showed that different molecular techniques applied to cytologic samples, such as FISH, quantitative polymerase chain reaction (PCR), and direct sequencing with fresh cells; scraped cells

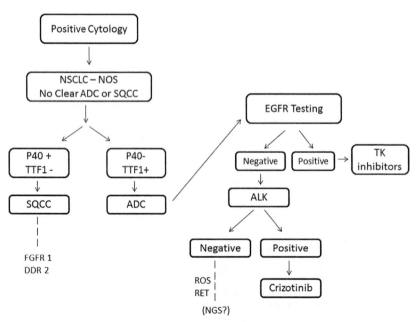

Fig. 4. Algorithm for use of ancillary techniques in NSCLC. *Abbreviations*: DDR, discoidin domain receptor family; FGFR, fibroblast growth factor receptor; NGS, next generation sequencing; RET, rearranged during transfection; ROS 1, c-ros oncogene 1.

from archival slides; and cell blocks have similar or higher accuracy and sensitivity compared with surgical specimens.[22]

Depending on the selection criteria, 10% to 20% of NSCLCs harbor EGFR mutations.[19] The most common oncogenic mutations in the tyrosine kinase domain of EGFR are small in-frame deletions in exon 19 and a point mutation (p.L858R) in exon 21 (**Fig. 5**).[4,17,23] Together these two mutations account for 80% to 90% of all EGFR mutations in NSCLCs.[19] Other mutations associated with response to TKIs include mutations in residues p.G719 (exon 18) and p.L861

(exon 21).[24] These mutations cause constitutive activation of EGFR and confer sensitivity to the TKIs gefinitib and erlotinib. Unfortunately, the effect of these drugs tends to be limited in time due to the emergence of drug resistance. A second mutation, T790M in exon 20, appears in approximately half of all patients with acquired resistance to TKIs. Besides selecting patients for treatment, the screening of EGFR mutations is used for detecting resistance mutations. The most common method of mutation detection — involving DNA purification from the tumor sample, PCR-based amplification, and sequencing — is

Fig. 5. Detection of the EGFR mutation p.L858R in DNA extracted from cytology material. Upper electropherogram: wild-type sequence. Lower electropherogram: mutated sequence.

EGFR mutation screening

	855					860		
Thr	Asp	Phe	Gly	Leu	Ala	Lys	Leu	Leu
Thr	Asp	Phe	Gly	Leu/Arg	Ala	Lys	Leu	Leu

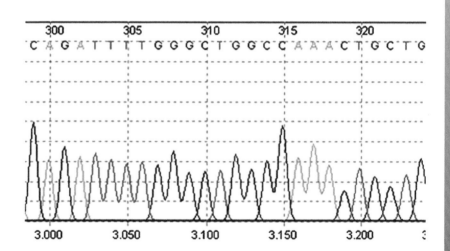

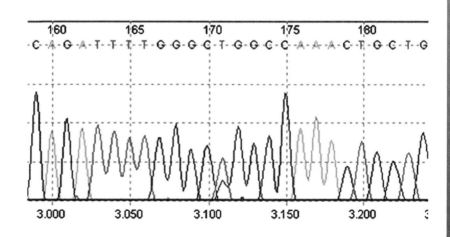

suitable for cytologic samples because it can use a limited number of tumor cells.

KRAS mutations are found in 30% of lung ADCs and 5% of SqCCs. The KRAS ADCs are mainly of the mucinous type and have been associated with smokers, KRAS and EGFR molecular alterations tend to be mutually exclusive, and patients with the KRAS mutation do not benefit from TKI therapy.[25] So at this stage, there seems to be little gain in including KRAS mutation testing in routine clinical practice. It is likely, however, that in the near future the inclusion of additional predictive markers in routine molecular testing will justify inclusion of KRAS testing as a negative predictive biomarker.

The rearrangement of the ALK gene with different gene partners, namely EML4, has recently been detected in approximately 5% of NSCLCs.[4] ALK and EML4 are both located on the short arm of chromosome 2 separated by 12 Mb and are oriented in opposite 5' to 3' directions. Two different variants of EML4-ALK fusion gene have been characterized, both involving exon 20 to 29 of ALK fused to exon 1 to 13 (variant 1) or exon 1 to 20 (variant 2) of EML4. Patients exhibiting tumors with ALK gene rearrangements are in general male and are resistant to EGFR inhibitors.[6] There is now a drug, PF-02341066- crizotinib (dual MET/ALK inhibitor), which inhibits this oncogene. ALK rearrangement-positive patients treated with the novel ALK inhibitor, crizotinib, showed an overall response rate of 57%, with 72% having a progression-free survival of 6 months or greater.[6] These EML4-ALK ADCs show lower levels of ALK protein than other neoplasms that are also associated with ALK mutations (anaplastic T-cell lymphoma). The determination of ALK protein expression by ICC or using fluorescence in situ hybridization (FISH) probes in EGFR-TKI–negative ADCs is fundamental for treatment and can be performed on cytologic material.[26]

It is important to encourage proper collection and handling of cytologic samples to validate these novel techniques in future prospective large patient cohort studies. Discrepancies in mutation status between primary tumors and corresponding metastases can appear, and these may have significant implication in TKI therapy for NSCLC patients. Studies on the clinical impact of discrepancies between primary and metastatic cancers, however, are still needed.

PRACTICAL APPLICATIONS

Specific therapies are selected for patients with lung cancer depending on the cytohistologic diagnosis and the molecular profile of the tumor. Currently, the recommendations for EGFR mutation testing and eligibility for pemetrexed or bevacizumab therapy are for lung cancers with a diagnosis of ADC; NSCLC, favor ADC; or NSCLC-NOS. For this reason, when confronting a tumor with an NSCLC morphology, the primary decision for a pathologist is whether the tumor is a definitive SqCC or NSCLC, favor ADC. On the other hand, when morphology or ICC findings are equivocal, pathologists need to keep in mind that a diagnosis of SqCC or NSCLC, favor SqCC excludes those patients from cytohistologically driven molecular testing or chemotherapy. In such a situation, it is better to favor NSCLC-NOS, to allow the patient eligibility for the therapeutic options available. This is why a TTF-1–negative tumor that is with weak or focal P63 stain should be classified as NSCLC-NOS rather than NSCLC, favor SqCC.[3]

For molecular testing, pathologists should use formalin-fixed, paraffin-embedded specimens or fresh frozen or alcohol-fixed specimens. As discussed previously, cytologic samples are suitable for molecular testing. In this case, cell blocks are preferred to smear preparations. The adequacy of specimens for molecular testing should be performed by a pathologist assessing cancer cell content. Although each laboratory should establish the minimum proportion of cancer cells needed for mutation detection during validation, in the authors' experience, molecular tests are able to detect DNA alterations in samples with as few as 20% tumor cells. When needed, microdissection or macrodissection for tumor cell enrichment could be performed. Different methodologies are available both for the detection of EGFR mutations and ALK rearrangements and, at this stage, no thorough comparison of these methods has been performed. With variable specifications for sensitivity and specificity, each laboratory has to validate its method of choice. In the authors' opinion, molecular testing methods should be able to detect the vast majority of individual mutations that have been reported in lung ADC. It is also important to remember that if a laboratory performs testing on specimens from patients with acquired resistance to EGFR kinase inhibitors, then those tests should be able to detect the secondary EGFR p.T790M mutation. In this case, the sensitivity needed for detecting mutated DNA molecules amidst wild-type molecules may increase significantly, and methods that are able to detect EGFR mutations in as few as 5% of tumor cells may be needed.

> ## Key Points
> ### PRACTICAL APPLICATIONS OF MOLECULAR TESTING
>
> 1. All patients with lung ADC should be tested for EGFR activating mutations and ALK rearrangements. Patients should not be excluded from testing based on clinical features.
>
> 2. EGFR mutation and ALK rearrangement testing should be ordered at the time of diagnosis for patients presenting with advanced stage or at time of recurrence/progression in patients who originally presented with lower-stage disease but were not previously tested.
>
> 3. Where an ADC component cannot be completely excluded, for example, due to limited cellularity (tissue biopsy or cytology), EGFR and ALK testing may be performed in cases showing squamous or small cell histology.
>
> 4. To determine EGFR and ALK status, primary or metastatic tumors are equally suitable for testing.
>
> 5. Pathologists should determine the specimen adequacy for EGFR testing by assessing cancer cell content. Laboratories may use any validated testing methods, but tests that are able to detect DNA alterations in samples with as few as 20% tumor cells are recommended. Microdissection for tumor cell enrichment should be performed when needed.

FUTURE TRENDS

Currently, genetic predictive biomarker evaluation in lung cancer is performed only once, mostly at the time of diagnosis. In the near future, it is likely that the study of such predictive biomarkers will be performed continuously with the purposes of monitoring disease progression, identifying the acquisition of therapy resistance mechanisms, and, consequently, leading to better informed therapy decisions. This wider use of predictive biomarkers is expected to be fueled by the development of new technologies (most notably next-generation sequencing) and by the furthering of understanding cancer cell survival mechanisms in NSCLC.

The increasing demand on tumor tissue for testing purposes will push forward optimization of currently available sample types as well as the concept of liquid biopsy in the clinical management of cancer patients. The possibility of identifying tumor-specific (somatic) mutations in blood that can serve as biomarkers for tumor detection, monitor tumor response to specific therapies, and detect residual disease after surgery and long-term follow-up, is highly attractive.[27] This is especially pertinent for tumors, such as NSCLC, for which access to tumor material is frequently limited. Although the intrinsic low abundance of circulating tumor cells and/or cell-free tumor DNA makes the detection and quantification of such mutations in blood a challenging task, there is a compelling body of evidence supporting the feasibility of such a task.[28] Again, technology

developments and better understanding of the molecular biology of NSCLC are of paramount importance in achieving those goals.

REFERENCES

1. Tani EM, Schmitt FC, Oliveira ML, et al. Pulmonary cytology in tuberculosis. Acta Cytol 1987; 31:460–3.

2. Rekhtman N, Brandt SM, Sigel CS, et al. Suitability of thoracic cytology for new therapeutic paradigms in non-small cell lung carcinoma: high accuracy of tumor subtyping and feasibility of EGFR and KRAS molecular testing. J Thorac Oncol 2011;6:451–8.

3. Travis WD, Brambilla E, Noguchi M, et al. Diagnosis of lung cancer in small biopsies and cytology. Implications of the 2011 International Association for the Study of Lung Cancer/American Thoracic Society/European Respiratory Society Classification. Arch Pathol Lab Med 2013;137:668–84.

4. Schmitt F, Barroca H. Role of ancillary studies in fine-needle aspiration from selected tumors. Cancer Cytopathol 2012;120:145–60.

5. Johnson DH, Fehrenbacher L, Novotny WF, et al. Randomized ohase II trial comparing bevacizumab plus carboplatin and paclitaxel with carboplatin and palicataxel alone in previously untreated locally advanced or metastatic non-small cell lung cancer. J Clin Oncol 2004;22:2184–91.

6. Kwak EL, Bang YJ, Camidge DR, et al. Anaplastic lymphoma kinase inhibition in non-small cell lung cancer. N Engl J Med 2010;363:1693–703.

7. Scagliotti G, Hanna N, Fossella F, et al. The differential efficacy of pemetrexed according to NSCLC

histology: a review of two Phase III studies. Oncologist 2009;14:253–63.

8. Silje Haukali O, Henrik H, Olsen EK, et al. Subtyping of nonsmall cell lung cancer on cytology specimens: reproducibility of cytopathologic diagnoses on sparse material. Diagn Cytopathol 2013. http://dx.doi.org/10.1002/dc.22995.

9. Kalhor N, Zander DS, Liu J. TTF-1 and P63 for distinguishing pulmonary small-cell carcinoma from poorly differentiated squamous cell carcinoma in previously pap-stained cytologic material. Mod Pathol 2006;19:1117–23.

10. Righi L, Graziano P, Fornari A, et al. Immunohistochemical subtyping of nonsmall cell lung cancer not otherwise specified in fine-needle aspiration cytology. Cancer 2011;117:3416–23.

11. Pelosi G, Fabbri A, Bianchi F, et al. ΔNp63 (p40) and thyroid transcription factor-1 immunoreactivity on small biopsies or cellblocks for typing non-small cell lung cancer. A novel two-hit sparing-material approach. J Thorac Oncol 2012;7:281–90.

12. Nobre A, Albergaria A, Schmitt F. P40: a p63 isoform useful for lung cancer diagnosis-A review of the physiological and pathological role of p63. Acta Cytol 2013;57:1–8.

13. Fatima N, Cohen C, Lawson D, et al. TTF1 and Napsin A double stain: a useful marker for diagnosing lung adenocarcinomas on fine-needle aspiration cell blocks. Cancer Cytopathol 2011;119:127–33.

14. Rekhtman N, Ang DC, Sima CS, et al. Immunohistochemical algorithm for differentiation of lung adenocarcinoma and squamous cell carcinoma based on large series of whole-tissue sections with validation in small specimens. Mod Pathol 2011;24:1348–59.

15. Yoshida A, Tsuta K, Watanabe S, et al. Frequent ALK rearrangement and TTF1/p63 co-expression in lung adenocarcinoma with signet-ring cell component. Lung Cancer 2011;72:309–15.

16. Travis WD, Brambilla E, Noguchi M, et al. International association for the study of lung cancer/American thoracic society/European respiratory society international multidisciplinary classification of lung adenocarcinoma. J Thorac Oncol 2011;6:244–85.

17. Ramalingam SS, Owonikoko TK, Khuri FR. Lung cancer: new biological insights and recent therapeutic advances. CA Cancer J Clin 2011;61:91–112.

18. Garassino MC, Borgonovo K, Rossi A, et al. Biological and clinical features in predicting efficacy of epidermal growth factor receptor tyrosine kinase inhibitors: a systematic review and meta-analysis. Anticancer Res 2009;29:2691–701.

19. Shepherd FA, Rodrigues Pereira J, Ciuleanu T, et al. Erlotinib in previously treated non-small-cell lung cancer. N Engl J Med 2005;353:123–32.

20. Stinchcombe TE, Socinski MA. Gefitinib in advanced non-small cell lung cancer: does it deserve a second chance? Oncologist 2008;13:933–44.

21. Thatcher N, Chang A, Parikh P, et al. Gefitinib plus best supportive care in previously treated patients with refractory advanced non-small-cell lung cancer: results from a randomised, placebo-controlled, multicentre study (Iressa Survival Evaluation in Lung Cancer). Lancet 2005;366:1527–37.

22. da Cunha Santos G, Saieg MA, Geddie W, et al. EGFR gene status in cytological samples of non-small cell lung carcinoma: controversies and opportunities. Cancer Cytopathol 2011. http://dx.doi.org/10.1002/cncy.20150.

23. Ding L, Getz G, Wheeler DA, et al. Somatic mutations affect key pathways in lung adenocarcinoma. Nature 2008;455:1069–75.

24. Greulich H, Chen TH, Feng W, et al. Oncogenic transformation by inhibitor-sensitive and resistant EGFR mutants. PLoS Med 2005;2(11):e313.

25. Billah S, Stewart J, Staerkel G, et al. EGFR and KRAS mutations in lung carcinoma: molecular testing by using cytology specimens. Cancer Cytopathol 2011. http://dx.doi.org/10.1002/cncy.20151.

26. Savic S, Bubendorf L. Role of fluorescence in situ hybridization in lung cancer cytology. Acta Cytol 2012;56:611–21.

27. Aparicio S, Caldas C. The implications of clonal genome evolution for cancer medicine. N Engl J Med 2013;368:842–51.

28. Kang Y, Pantel K. Tumor cell dissemination: emerging biological insights from animal models and cancer patients. Cancer Cell 2013;23:573–81.

Ancillary Studies in Thyroid Cytopathology

N. Paul Ohori, MD*, Karen E. Schoedel, MD

KEYWORDS

- Thyroid • Neoplasm • Molecular pathology • *BRAF* • *RAS* • *RET/PTC* • *PAX8/PPAR*γ • *Veracyte*
- *Afirma*

ABSTRACT

Recent advances in thyroid imaging, clinical evaluation, cytopathology, surgical pathology, and molecular diagnostics have contributed toward greater understanding of thyroid nodules. In particular, the development of the Bethesda System for Reporting Thyroid Cytopathology (BSRTC) has brought standardization to the field and the system dovetails well with the implementation of immunohistochemistry and molecular testing to diagnostic practice. Among the molecular strategies available, the application of the molecular panel of common genetic alterations can stratify indeterminate BSRTC diagnoses into low-risk and high-risk groups. The molecular panel markers have a high positive predictive value and therefore, the panel is considered to be a "rule-in" test. In contrast, the Afirma gene expression classifier by Veracyte Corporation is a test that has been reported to have a high negative predictive value, and therefore, considered to be a "rule-out" test. With further advances, refinements are expected to be made. In particular, the application of next-generation sequencing technology holds promise in bringing thyroid cytopathology to the next level.

OVERVIEW

Fine needle aspiration (FNA) cytology has proven to be an effective method for collecting material that provides characteristics of thyroid nodules and estimates the risk of malignancy. Over recent decades, refinements have been made in imaging, localization of lesions, sampling technique, specimen processing, standardized reporting, and application of ancillary studies. In particular, advances in thyroid molecular testing have taken place in parallel with the implementation of a standardized reporting system for classifying thyroid FNA samples: the Bethesda System for Reporting Thyroid Cytopathology (BSRTC).[1,2] In this review, we provide an overview of how recent developments in clinical molecular testing have impacted the evaluation of thyroid nodules. First, we discuss the common differential diagnoses associated with the BSRTC categories. Then, we focus on the application of ancillary testing to thyroid cytopathology, in particular the use of immunohistochemistry (IHC) and molecular testing in common follicular-derived thyroid neoplasms. Recent correlation studies have shed light on the association of BSRTC diagnoses with certain molecular alterations and outcome. This knowledge provides powerful insight into predicting the nature of the thyroid nodule. However, to determine the best management strategy from the cytopathologic and molecular information, the findings should be interpreted in the appropriate context to avoid pitfalls. Finally, we mention some technologies that may influence future trends in this area.

Financial Disclosures: The authors have no disclosures.
Department of Pathology, University of Pittsburgh Medical Center-Presbyterian, A610, 200 Lothrop Street, Pittsburgh, PA 15213, USA
* Corresponding author.
E-mail address: ohorinp@upmc.edu

Surgical Pathology 7 (2014) 47–60
http://dx.doi.org/10.1016/j.path.2013.10.001

surgpath.theclinics.com

DIFFERENTIAL DIAGNOSIS ASSOCIATED WITH BSRTC CATEGORIES

One of the main challenges in thyroid cytopathology stems from the fact that a significant proportion of malignancies are low-grade follicular-derived carcinomas with cytopathologic features that overlap with benign hyperplastic or neoplastic nodules.[3] Furthermore, thyroid FNAs have a low pretest probability of malignancy (approximately 5%–10%). These features contribute to the placement of 20% to 30% of cases in one of the indeterminate BSRTC diagnoses (atypia of undetermined significance/follicular lesion of undetermined significance [AUS/FLUS], follicular neoplasm/suspicious for follicular neoplasm [FN/SFN], and suspicious for malignancy [SMC]). The remaining cases are placed in the benign (50%–70%), malignant (4%–8%), and unsatisfactory/nondiagnostic (10%–20%) categories. The demarcations between the categories are not always clear and are influenced by a variety of factors, including FNA sampling technique and yield, specimen processing, threshold for reporting cytologic atypia, interobserver variability in histopathologic interpretation of the resected nodule, tolerance of false-negative diagnoses, and methods used to calculate risk of malignancy.[4]

Some variability in practice is inevitable. Nonetheless, the BSRTC categories and subcategories (based on specific architectural and cytologic features) are associated with sets of differential diagnoses, depending on specific cytologic features identified (Table 1). For the benign diagnosis, the bland cytologic features of cellular elements usually ensure a benign outcome. However, some FNAs may sample focal areas of malignancies that, in part, are composed of deceptively bland-appearing neoplastic cells. In particular, large follicular variant papillary thyroid carcinoma (FVPTC) with macrofollicular areas and patchy distribution of diagnostic nuclear features may escape detection. Therefore, diagnostic scrutiny is warranted, especially for large nodules. The differential diagnosis for the AUS/FLUS diagnosis depends on the type of atypia identified: cytologic nuclear atypia (falling short of the "suspicious for malignancy" [SMC] diagnosis), architectural atypia (falling short of the "follicular neoplasm/suspicious for follicular neoplasm" [FN/SFN] diagnosis) or both. The FN/SFN cases are usually hypercellular specimens that do not show overt cytologic features of malignancy but are predominantly composed of microfollicles and/or syncytia; these cases reveal outcome possibilities including nodular hyperplasia, follicular adenoma (FA), follicular carcinoma (FC), FVPTC, and PTC with focal microfollicular pattern. Because the cytologic diagnosis of malignancy usually is based on nuclear details, the SMC and positive for malignancy (PMC) diagnoses share similar differential diagnoses. FC and cases of FVPTC in which the nuclear details are subtle would not be considered in the differential diagnosis of SMC or PMC.

Bethesda System for Reporting Thyroid Cytopathology diagnostic categories with cancer risk and recommended management		
Category	Cancer Risk (%)	Recommended Management Based on Bethesda Guidelines
Unsatisfactory/Nondiagnostic	1–4	Repeat fine-needle aspiration (FNA)
Benign	0–3	Clinical follow-up
Atypia of undetermined significance/follicular lesion of undetermined significance	5–15 (for initial diagnosis) 20–25 (for repeat diagnosis)	Repeat FNA Consider lobectomy
Follicular neoplasm/suspicious for follicular neoplasm	15–30	Lobectomy
Suspicious for malignancy	60–77	Lobectomy or total thyroidectomy
Positive for malignancy	97–99	Total thyroidectomy

Data from Ali SZ. Thyroid cytopathology: Bethesda and beyond. Acta Cytol 2011;55:4–12.

Table 1
Differential diagnosis of BSRTC categories and major outcomes in consideration

BSRTC Category	Specific Feature(s)	Differential Diagnosis Regarding Outcome
Benign	Colloid nodule	• Nodular hyperplasia • Macrofollicular areas from FA, FC, FVPTC (rare)
	Lymphocytic thyroiditis	• Lymphocytic thyroiditis • Lymphoma • PTC (vs oncocytic cells with atypia) (rare)
	Follicular nodule with hyperplastic features	• Graves disease • FA, FC, FVPTC, PTC (rare)
	Granulomas	• Subacute thyroiditis • Infection • Reaction to neoplasm
AUS/FLUS	Cytologic atypia	• Nodular hyperplasia with reactive change • FA with atypia • FC • FVPTC • PTC • Other neoplasms
	Architectural atypia (microfollicles present)	• Nodular hyperplasia with microfollicles • FA • FC • FVPTC • PTC (with focal microfollicular pattern) • Other neoplasms/lesions (eg, parathyroid)
	Cytologic and architectural atypia	• Nodular hyperplasia • FA • FC • FVPTC • PTC (with focal microfollicular pattern) • Other neoplasms
FN/SFN	Cellular microfollicular predominant sample	• Nodular hyperplasia with microfollicles • FA • FC • FVPTC • PTC (with focal microfollicular pattern) • Other neoplasms/lesions (eg, parathyroid)
SMC	Highly atypical cells (but not diagnostic of malignancy)	• PTC • FVPTC • MTC • PDC • AC • Lymphoma • Metastasis Less likely considerations • Oncocytic neoplasms/lesions • Other reactive changes

(continued on next page)

Table 1
(Continued)

BSRTC Category	Specific Feature(s)	Differential Diagnosis Regarding Outcome
Malignant	Features depend on particular neoplasm	• PTC • FVPTC (if nuclear features are present) • MTC • PDC • AC • Metastasis Avoid • Oncocytic neoplasms/lesions • Other reactive changes

Abbreviations: AC, anaplastic carcinoma; AUS/FLUS, atypia of undetermined significance/follicular lesion of undetermined significance; BSRTC, Bethesda System for Reporting Thyroid Cytopathology; FAd, follicular adenoma; FCa, follicular carcinoma; FN/SFN, follicular neoplasm/suspicious for follicular neoplasm; FV, follicular variant; MTC, medullary thyroid carcinoma; PDC, poorly differentiated carcinoma; PTC, papillary thyroid carcinoma; SMC, suspicious for malignancy.

ANCILLARY STUDIES

IMMUNOHISTOCHEMISTRY

Immunohistochemistry (IHC) is being used with increasing frequency in cytopathology and at certain institutions is contributing significantly to the diagnostic interpretation of thyroid nodules. In contrast to the use of IHC for standard formalin-fixed paraffin-embedded histology tissue, the application of IHC to cytology specimens requires additional attention to detail. IHC on thyroid cytology specimens may be performed on a variety of preparations: cell blocks, liquid-based cytology specimens, and direct smears. Each type of preparation has its own advantages and disadvantages.[5] Because cell block preparations are virtually identical to small biopsy paraffin blocks, the IHC staining protocol and controls may be performed similarly to traditional methods in surgical pathology. The main disadvantage is the inability to determine the cellularity of the cell block material at the time of specimen collection (even with immediate on-site evaluation) resulting in hypocellular and insufficient cell block material for IHC in a subset of cases. IHC may be applied to liquid-based cytology specimens that are derived from FNA sources and its efficacy has been demonstrated.[6,7] Performing IHC on this type of specimen has the advantage of optimal cell preservation, elimination of obscuring background, and reasonable shelf-life of the specimen in liquid preservative for up to 6 to 8 weeks. Multiple "blank" slides for IHC may be produced from the stored tissue specimen in liquid preservative.

However, the standard IHC staining protocol used for histologic paraffin blocks may need to be modified. Moreover, a histologic paraffin block section may not serve as an appropriate positive control. On the other hand, the ideal positive control specimen in liquid preservative may not be readily available, and producing a control slide may be a challenge. In addition to the specimen types mentioned previously, air-dried direct smears may be used for IHC. For using direct smears, foresight and planning are required for ideal results. The initial slides may be stained by Diff-Quik, for example, to confirm the quality and quantity of the lesional cell population. If multiple IHC stains are anticipated, blank smears on positively charged slides may be prepared from the FNA specimen.[5] The IHC staining protocol may require modification of that used for histologic paraffin blocks and performing positive controls would require having stored blank smears with tissue appropriate for the IHC stain. Negative controls would require having a blank test smear.

The major role of IHC is its use as a differentiation marker. In thyroid cytopathology, the most important uses involve the diagnoses of medullary carcinoma, parathyroid neoplasms, lymphoma, and metastases. Therefore, IHC markers, such as calcitonin, carcinoembryonic antigen (CEA), thyroid transcription factor-1, thyroglobulin, PAX-8, parathyroid hormone, a variety of lymphoid markers, and organ site–related markers (eg, carbonic anhydrase IX for renal cell carcinoma) are useful. For example, a cellular population of single cells and cell aggregates (but not characteristically microfollicular in pattern) without obvious nuclear features of PTC or medullary carcinoma may be considered for the possibility of a primary or metastatic neoplasm. The differential diagnosis may include FVPTC, solid variant of PTC, follicular carcinoma, poorly differentiated carcinoma, medullary carcinoma, parathyroid neoplasm, and metastases, such as carcinoma from the breast or lung. In such cases, a reasonable panel of IHC stains to address the differentiation of the cell population would include thyroid transcription factor-1, thyroglobulin, PAX-8, calcitonin, CEA, parathyroid hormone, Napsin-A, and Gross Cystic Disease Fluid Protein (GCDFP).

IHC also has a potential use in establishing a malignant diagnosis in cytopathology. In rare reports, IHC markers, such as HBME-1, CK19, and Galectin-3, have been shown to demonstrate relatively high sensitivity and specificity for the diagnosis of carcinoma in thyroid cytology samples. The individual sensitivities of these markers ranged from 75% to 100% and the specificities ranged from 70.5% to 95.0%.[8–10] In light of sampling issues and the focal immunoreactivity, tumor marker IHC is used more effectively in resection specimens. However, even with ample tissue specimen, the low specificities of some immunostains imply relatively high false positivity and, therefore, these immunostains should be used and interpreted with caution. Moreover, the mechanism of how the epitopes of antibodies are involved in carcinogenesis is not clear. For example, HBME-1 is an antibody generated against the microvilli of mesothelial cells and, therefore, the expected immunoreactivity is seen along the cell membranes.[11] Some investigators have found that the combined positivity of markers such as HBME-1 and CK19 provides enhanced sensitivity and specificity.[8] Whether or not these immunostains are sufficiently robust to be used in routine practice would need to be tested and determined by individual laboratories.

More recently, the application of mutation-specific markers has drawn much attention. In particular, detection of the *BRAF* V600E mutation by IHC holds promise, especially because this mutation is involved in thyroid carcinogenesis (see later in this article). Studies to date have been conducted on resected thyroid surgical pathology and tissue microarray specimens.[12–15] These studies show that the mutation-specific *BRAF* V600E antibody correlates well with the actual mutation, as demonstrated by direct sequencing and mass spectrometry genotyping assay. Evaluation of staining intensity appears to be valuable, because only the strong IHC staining is specific for the *BRAF* V600E mutation. Although cytology-based studies using this antibody are forthcoming, this technique is most likely adaptable to FNA thyroid cytology specimens because the staining pattern of positive cases is diffuse and homogeneous, thus minimizing the possibility of sampling error.[15] Furthermore, cases with positive *BRAF* V600E IHC results and negative mutation results may raise the question of "false-negative" molecular results, as a large number of non-neoplastic cells in low tumor density samples may dilute the small number of neoplastic cells.[13]

MOLECULAR TESTING

The application of molecular testing has the potential to add another dimension to the evaluation of thyroid FNA specimens. Because the benign and malignant diagnoses have high negative predictive value (NPV) and positive predictive value (PPV), respectively, the main contribution of molecular testing pertains to the indeterminate diagnoses, in particular the AUS/FLUS and FN/SFN diagnoses. Over the past few years, studies have investigated the role of molecular testing in cytopathology. In this regard, 2 main approaches have been developed. The first involves the application of a "molecular panel of common genetic alterations" to indeterminate samples. This type of test has been investigated at independent academic institutions[16–18] and is available as a commercial test (miRInform, Asuragen, Austin, TX). The molecular panel approach has high PPV and

---

IHC markers in thyroid cytopathology

Differentiation Markers
- Thyroid transcription factor-1
- Thyroglobulin
- PAX-8
- Calcitonin
- CEA
- Parathyroid hormone
- Napsin-A
- GCDFP

Associated Tumor Markers
- HBME-1
- CK19
- Galectin-3

Mutation-Specific Marker
- *BRAF* V600E

is therefore, a "rule-in" test; it also provides information on lesional characteristics. However, a negative molecular test by the current molecular panel result does not exclude malignancy, although the risk is decreased significantly. The second approach involves the gene expression classifier, which is represented by the *Afirma* test by Vercyte Corporation (South San Francisco, CA). This test evaluates the mRNA expression of 167 genes in thyroid samples and is designed as a "rule-out" test by having a high NPV.

MOLECULAR PANEL OF COMMON GENETIC ALTERATIONS IN THYROID NEOPLASMS

The molecular panel approach is based on the fact that more than 70% of common thyroid neoplasms (PTC, FC, FA, poorly differentiated carcinoma [PDC], and anaplastic carcinoma [AC]) demonstrate one of the molecular alterations (*BRAF, RAS, RET/PTC,* and *PAX 8/PPARγ*) involving the mitogen-activated protein kinase (MAPK) pathway.[19] These genetic alterations are, for the most part, mutually exclusive of each other and application of molecular testing to cytology specimens has the potential to detect point mutations or gene rearrangements in samples in which neoplastic cells show subtle cytologic changes or in samples in which the neoplastic cells are not well represented. For detection of point mutations (*BRAF, RAS*), the molecular samples may be collected from fresh specimens or fixed tissue for polymerase chain reaction (PCR)-based detection of point mutations.[16] On the other hand, for translocations/gene rearrangements (*RET/PTC, PAX 8/PPARγ*), molecular samples ideally are obtained from fresh specimens for RNA isolation (and subsequent reverse-transcriptase PCR of translocation points) or from fixed cells on glass slides (eg, cell block, monolayer preparations) for fluorescence in-situ hybridization (FISH). The preference of methods depends on the laboratory and molecular pathologists at the individual institution.

BRAF

BRAF mutation of the V600E type is the most common *BRAF* mutation and has a cancer risk of more than 99%.[2] Similarly, the specificity of *BRAF* V600E mutation is more than 99%. This mutation is found in approximately 45% of PTC and most of these neoplasms are the classic-type or tall-cell variant (TCV) and much less frequently FVPTC. Although most adequately cellular FNA specimens from classic PTC and TCV PTC show robust nuclear changes (nuclear grooves and pseudoinclusions), some samples may represent areas of the neoplasm with more subtle nuclear changes.

Therefore, a *BRAF* V600E mutation in the context of an indeterminate cytology diagnosis is informative and has the potential to influence clinical management.[16] *BRAF* V600E mutation is seen also in poorly differentiated carcinoma and anaplastic carcinoma. Other types of *BRAF* mutation, most notably the K601E type, are found in 1% to 2% of PTCs. Thyroid neoplasms with the *BRAF* K601E mutation show different cytologic and pathologic features in contrast to *BRAF* V600E-mutated PTC.[20] *BRAF* K601E-mutated PTCs demonstrate follicular or microfollicular growth pattern and are diagnosed as FVPTC or rarely as FC or FA.[20–22]

RAS

RAS mutations in the thyroid (usually *NRAS61* or *HRAS61* mutation and less commonly *KRAS 12/13* mutation) are associated with follicular patterned lesions with encapsulation and lack of lymph node metastases.[23] This mutation has a positive predictive value of 74% to 87% for malignancy and the differential diagnosis includes FVPTC, FC, FA, PDC, AC, and rarely hyperplastic nodules.[16–18] The vast majority of benign nodules with *RAS* mutation are FAs, which have been shown to have this mutation in approximately 30% of cases. Because the *RAS* mutation is found in both well-differentiated and poorly differentiated/anaplastic carcinomas, it most likely represents an early event in thyroid carcinogenesis.

RET/PTC

Clonal *RET/PTC* chromosomal rearrangement has specificity of greater than 99% for malignancy and is found in 10% to 20% of PTC cases.[2,19] *RET/PTC1* and *RET/PTC3* are the most common subtypes that are associated with adult cases with radiation exposure (mostly classic PTC histologic type) and pediatric cases with radiation exposure (solid PTC histologic type), respectively. In contrast to PTC cases with *BRAF* V600E or *RAS* mutation, *RET/PTC*-rearranged PTC cases show a favorable prognosis and usually do not progress to PDC or AC.

PAX 8/PPARγ

PAX 8/PPARγ gene rearrangement involves the translocation of the *PAX8* gene to the *PPARγ* gene in chromosomes 2 and 3, respectively. Initially, *PAX 8/PPARγ* translocated cases were closely associated with FC, although more recent studies have identified this marker in FA and FVPTC.[2] Thyroid neoplasms with *PAX 8/PPARγ* gene rearrangement are often smaller, associated with a microfollicular or solid histologic pattern, have a thick capsule, and demonstrate vascular/capsular invasion. This translocation has specificity of greater than 90% for malignancy and most benign cases are diagnosed as FA. Although approximately 8% of FA cases have been reported to demonstrate *PAX 8/PPARγ* gene rearrangement, attention to histologic detail is required for accurate classification of these cases. Some cases initially thought to have intact capsules have been shown to demonstrate capsular or vascular invasion after additional histologic sections were submitted.[19] Therefore, identification of this marker should prompt extensive histologic search for vascular and/or capsular invasion.

Other Molecular Alterations

TRK rearrangement is identified in a small percentage of PTC in some parts to the world.[19] Because of its low prevalence, the clinical significance is yet to be determined. Neoplasms dedifferentiating to PDC and AC demonstrate *p53* or *CTNNB1* (Betacatenin) point mutation in a significant proportion of cases. These mutations are thought to be late events because they are rarely found in PTC or FC.

the evaluation of thyroid nodules. However, testing of all samples is neither cost-effective nor reasonable, as most thyroid FNA specimens are benign. Therefore, these tests are best applied to the AUS/FLUS and FN/SFN diagnoses. Recent studies have shed light into the correlation of the BSRTC diagnoses, the typical molecular alterations, and expected outcomes.[20,23–25] The molecular test results may provide insight into the underlying reasons for indeterminate diagnoses, whether they are due to sampling, technical issues, nonspecific nuclear features, or tumor heterogeneity. Furthermore, molecular testing may be applied to the SMC and PMC diagnoses, not for diagnostic purposes, but for management purposes, as these mutations, such as *BRAF* V600E, are associated with lymph node metastasis, and the surgeon may choose to perform central compartment lymph node dissection at the time of thyroidectomy. Therefore, cytopathologists can play a critical role in interpreting the multifaceted findings for their clinical colleagues (Table 2).

AUS/FLUS cases may demonstrate architectural atypia but fall short of the FN/SFN diagnosis or demonstrate cytologic nuclear atypia but fall

Key ancillary tests: prevalence of common molecular alterations in thyroid neoplasms					
Molecular Alteration	PTC	FC	FA	PDC	AC
BRAF V600E	45% Overall 60% Classic 80% TCV 10% FV	—	—	15%	38%
BRAF K601	1%–2% (predominantly FVPTC)	Rare	Rare	—	—
N,H,K RAS	10%–20% (predominantly FVPTC)	40%–50%	7%–30%	25%–30%	40%–50%
RET/PTC 1	7%–14%	—	—	—	—
RET/PTC 3	3%–6%	—	—	—	—
PAX8/PPARγ	1%–5%	30%–35%	2%–13%	—	—
TRK	<5%	—	—	—	—
CTNNB1	—	—	—	10%–20%	60%–70%
p53	—	—	—	20%–30%	50%–80%

Abbreviations: AC, anaplastic carcinoma; FA, follicular adenoma; FC, follicular carcinoma; FV, follicular variant; PDC, poorly differentiated carcinoma; PTC, papillary thyroid carcinoma; TCV, tall-cell variant.

PRACTICAL APPLICATION OF MOLECULAR PANEL TESTING

Given the characteristics of the common mutational alterations described previously, application of molecular testing provides further insight into

short of the SMC diagnosis. The presence of molecular alterations provides clues into the characteristics of the underlying nodule. For example, a *BRAF* V600E mutation suggests partial sampling of classic PTC or TCV PTC (**Fig. 1**). In other words, better sampling may have yielded lesional cells

Table 2
Practical applications: BSRTC diagnosis, associated molecular alteration, and usual outcome

BSRTC Diagnosis	Molecular Alteration	Usual Outcome
AUS/FLUS	*BRAF V600E*	PTC, classic, or TCV
		FVPTC (rare)
	BRAF K601E	FVPTC
	N,H,K RAS	FVPTC
		FC
		Medullary carcinoma
		FA
		Hyperplastic nodule
	PAX8/PPARγ	FVPTC
FN/SFN	*N,H,K RAS*	FVPTC
		PTC, classic
		FC
		Medullary carcinoma
		FA
		Hyperplastic nodule
	BRAF K601	FVPTC
	BRAF V600E (rare)	PTC, classic
		FVPTC
SMC	*BRAF V600E*	PTC, classic
		FVPTC
		PTC, Warthin-like (rare)
	PAX8/PPARγ	FC
	N,H,K RAS	FVPTC
		FC
		FA
	RET/PTC	PTC, classic
Malignant	*BRAF V600E*	PTC, classic, or TCV
		FVPTC (rare)
		PTC, oncocytic (rare)
		AC
	N,H,K RAS (rare)	FVPTC
		Medullary carcinoma
		AC

Abbreviations: AC, anaplastic carcinoma; AUS/FLUS, atypia of undetermined significance/follicular lesion of undetermined significance; BSRTC, Bethesda System for Reporting Thyroid Cytopathology; FA, follicular adenoma; FC, follicular carcinoma; FN/SFN, follicular neoplasm/suspicious for follicular neoplasm; FV, follicular variant; PDC, poorly differentiated carcinoma; PTC, papillary thyroid carcinoma; SMC, suspicious for malignancy; TCV, tall-cell variant.

with diagnostic nuclear features of PTC. However, one should note that *BRAF* V600E mutation is not specific for PTC and may be found in other nonthyroid neoplasms, such as colonic and pulmonary adenocarcinoma, melanoma, and lymphoma. Other mutations, such as *BRAF* K601E mutation, *RAS* mutation, or *PAX 8/PPARγ* gene rearrangement in the context of AUS/FLUS cases with architectural atypia are associated frequently with the outcome of "follicular-patterned" neoplasms (FVPTC, FC, FA) (Fig. 2). As expected, similar associations are true regarding these mutations in FN/SFN cases. Pitfalls for these cases include the presence of *RAS* mutation in rare cases of nodular hyperplasia and medullary carcinoma. For SMC cases, the presence of any mutation usually is associated with PTC.

In addition to the qualitative associations between the indeterminate diagnoses and molecular test results, probabilistic information has been derived from a large-scale study of more than 1000 indeterminate cytology cases.[16] For these cases, a negative molecular test result by a panel of markers (*BRAF, RAS, RET/PTC,* and *PAX*

Pitfalls: cytomorphologic and molecular features		
Category	Pitfall	Issue
Cytomorphologic	Subtle nuclear changes in a background with abundant colloid	Avoid false-negative result. Tumor heterogeneity, especially in >4-cm nodules. Molecular testing in borderline cases may be informative.
	Rare intranuclear pseudoinclusions	Avoid false-positive result (eg, oncocytic adenoma/hyperplasia). Avoid false classification (eg, medullary carcinoma, metastasis).
Molecular	RAS mutations in benign hyperplastic nodules	The presence of RAS mutations is well documented in thyroid adenoma. However, on rare occasions, RAS mutations may be seen in benign hyperplastic nodules also.
	BRAF V600E positivity in other neoplasms	BRAF V600E mutation may be seen in colonic adenocarcinoma, pulmonary adenocarcinoma, malignant melanoma, and lymphoma.
	PAX8/PPARγ in "follicular adenoma"	Beware of making a follicular adenoma diagnosis in the context of PAX8/PPARγ translocation. Multiple sections may be required to demonstrate capsular/vascular invasion (for follicular carcinoma) or nuclear features (for papillary carcinoma).
	Regional/geographic differences in distribution of molecular alterations among thyroid neoplasms (when compared to North America)	Papillary carcinoma from East Asia appears to show a much higher incidence of BRAF mutation with different subtype correlation and behavior. Incidence of RAS and PAX8/PPARγ positive follicular carcinoma may be higher in Europe.
	Interpretation of mutation-negative cases	Even with a negative mutation result, an indeterminate cytology diagnosis still carries a risk for malignancy.

8/PPARγ) on AUS/FLUS, FN/SFN, and SMC cases decreased the risk of malignancy to 6%, 14%, and 28%, respectively. In contrast, a positive molecular test result by any of the markers increased the risk of malignancy to 88%, 87%, and 95%, respectively (Table 3).

THERAPEUTIC AND PROGNOSTIC APPLICATIONS OF MOLECULAR PANEL

The dichotomization of indeterminate cases into low-risk and high-risk groups by the molecular test panel can be clinically helpful in optimizing management.[26] Given the high probability of carcinoma in indeterminate cases with molecular test result positivity, the patient and the surgeon may consider up-front total thyroidectomy when one of the molecular markers is positive.[16,26] This approach obviates the need to perform a completion contralateral lobectomy, which is advised when malignancy is detected. Furthermore, an up-front total thyroidectomy for these cases reduces the risk of recurrent laryngeal nerve injury and has been shown to be cost effective.[27]

Of the molecular markers in the panel, RAS mutation has the lowest PPV of 74% to 87% for malignancy.[16–18] Although most benign RAS-mutated nodules are FA, some studies have shown that these neoplasms may be prone to malignant transformation. Therefore, resection of these nodules may have long-term survival benefits.[28–31] The decision for type of surgery and clinical management also may be influenced by the detection of BRAF V600E mutation, which is associated with aggressive clinico-pathologic features in PTC (eg, extrathyroidal extension, lymph node metastasis, tumor

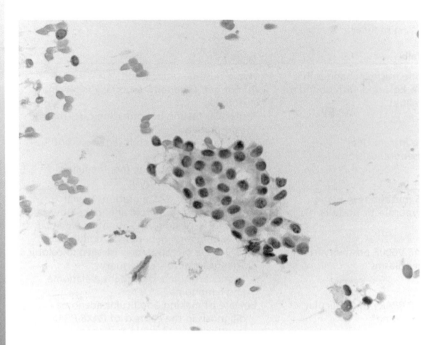

Fig. 1. AUS/FLUS case showing mild nuclear atypia. Molecular test showed *BRAF* V600E mutation and the resection outcome was a classic PTC. The cytology specimen represents partial sampling of the more subtle areas of PTC (Papanicolaou Stain, × 400).

recurrence, and mortality). These patients may benefit from total thyroidectomy and central compartment lymph node dissection.[26]

By the current panel of molecular tests (*BRAF, RAS, RET/PTC,* and *PAX 8/PPAR*γ) available, a positive molecular test result is highly informative and indicates high risk for malignancy. On the other hand, a negative molecular result in the context of an indeterminate diagnosis still carries a low risk for malignancy.[16] Further investigation and progress are needed for ancillary tests that would have higher NPV.

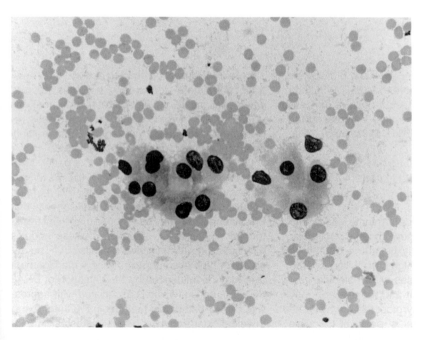

Fig. 2. AUS/FLUS case with focal microfollicle formation. Molecular test showed *NRAS61* mutation and the resection outcome was FVPTC (Diff-Quik Stain, × 400).

Table 3
BSRTC diagnostic categories and management options

BSRTC Diagnosis	Molecular Alteration (BRAF, RAS, RET/PTC, or PAX8/PPARγ)	Cancer Risk After Molecular Testing (%)	Management Options
AUS/FLUS	Negative	6	Observation vs repeat FNA vs lobectomy
	Positive	88	Total thyroidectomy
FN/SFN	Negative	14	Lobectomy
	Positive	87	Total thyroidectomy
SMC	Negative	28	Lobectomy
	Positive	95	Total thyroidectomy
PMC	Negative	>98	Total thyroidectomy
	Positive for any marker except BRAF V600E	>99	Total thyroidectomy
	BRAF V600E positive	>99	Total thyroidectomy and central lymph node dissection

Abbreviations: AUS/FLUS, atypia of undetermined significance/follicular lesion of undetermined significance; FN/SFN, follicular neoplasm/suspicious for follicular neoplasm; PMC, positive for malignancy; SMC, suspicious for malignancy.

AFIRMA GENE EXPRESSION CLASSIFIER

In contrast to the molecular panel of common genetic alterations, the gene expression classifier (GEC) approach focuses on the use of molecular testing as a "rule-out" test to identify cases with low probability of malignancy, in thyroid nodules with indeterminate diagnoses. This type of test is commercially available as the *Afirma* gene expression classifier by Veracyte Corporation.

The *Afirma* test system analyzes the genetic signatures of thyroid nodules by using a proprietary algorithm. It evaluates the expression of 167 genes: 25 genes to exclude rare lesions (such as melanoma, renal cell carcinoma, breast carcinoma, parathyroid tissue, and medullary carcinoma) and 142 genes to classify indeterminate thyroid nodules. Veracyte-sponsored studies have documented the analytical validity of the *Afirma* test, and demonstrated very high intranodule, intra-assay, interassay, and interlaboratory reproducibility (R^2 coefficients of 0.952, 0.988, 0.979, and 0.981, respectively).[32,33] Because the test requires shipment of molecular specimens to the testing site, the effect of specimen storage and varying shipping temperatures were tested and not shown to have any significant influence on the outcome of the GEC scores.

Clinical validation of the *Afirma* test was tested and documented in a recent study by Alexander et al,[34] wherein the "benign" *Afirma* test result was reported to have NPVs of 95%, 94%, and 85% for the AUS/FLUS, FN/SFN, and SMC indeterminate diagnoses. To place these figures into perspective, it is important to understand that NPVs and PPVs are influenced by the prevalence of disease in the cohort. The latter is particularly relevant for AUS/FLUS diagnosis, which has been shown to demonstrate interinstitutional variability in the outcome of malignancy.[4] Regarding the *Afirma* test, the NPV of 95% for the AUS/FLUS diagnosis is found in the context of 24% prevalence of malignancy. If the prevalence of malignancy for the AUS/FLUS diagnosis is lower in the test population, the NPV would be expected to increase. The purportedly high NPV of the *Afirma* test is its strength, which allows the recommendation of managing the indeterminate cytology cases (AUS/FLUS, FN/SFN) with "benign" *Afirma* test result to be treated comparably with benign cytology cases. By comparison, the 94% NPV of the molecular panel (BRAF, RAS, RET/PTC, and PAX 8/PPARγ) for the AUS/FLUS diagnosis is seen in the setting of 14% prevalence of malignancy. If one extrapolates the molecular test panel data to the 24% prevalence of malignancy as seen in the *Afirma* study, the NPV of the molecular panel test would drop to 89%.[35]

PRACTICAL APPLICATIONS OF THE *AFIRMA* GEC TEST

The molecular panel (BRAF, RAS, RET/PTC, and PAX 8/PPARγ) is designed as a "rule-in" test with a high PPV (74%–99% depending on the marker) as discussed previously. In this regard, the *Afirma* test has PPVs of only 38%, 37%, and 76% for the AUS/FLUS, FN/SFN, and SMC diagnoses, respectively.[32] Furthermore, a study by Duick et al,[36] showed that 52.3%, 10.5%, and 37.2% of *Afirma* GEC tests on cytologically indeterminate cases resulted in molecularly "benign," "inadequate," and "suspicious" classifications, respectively. These results suggest that for approximately one-half of tested cases (molecularly "inadequate" and "suspicious"), the *Afirma* test results may be questionable in value. Overall, the effectiveness of the molecular test appears to be in part dependent on the prevalence of malignancy associated with each indeterminate diagnosis. The strength of the *Afirma* GEC test is the weakness of the molecular panel (*BRAF, RAS, RET/PTC,* and *PAX 8/PPARγ*) and vice versa.

In addition to the predictive values and statistical analyses, clinical application of the *Afirma* study has some qualitative differences worth noting. Twenty (11%) of the 180 benign thyroid nodules were classified as "follicular tumor of uncertain malignant potential" or "well-differentiated tumor of uncertain malignant potential."[34] These diagnoses are not listed the current World Health Organization histologic classification of thyroid tumors[37] and are not likely to be used at many institutions. Furthermore, institutions that choose to dichotomize their tumors into adenomas and carcinomas may place some of these "tumors of uncertain malignant potential" into the malignant category. Given the degree of interobserver variability that exists in the histologic interpretation of thyroid nodules,[38] prediction of how these cases would be interpreted at other institutions is difficult to make. Nonetheless, variability in the histologic interpretation of thyroid nodules may have a significant impact on the negative predictive value of the *Afirma* test, as well as other ancillary tests.

In theory, the concept and technology behind the *Afirma* test are very attractive and potentially useful. However, the vast majority of publications on the *Afirma* test have been authored or coauthored by investigators affiliated with Veracyte Corporation.[32–36,39,40] A number of questions remain to be answered by larger case series performed by independent nonindustry-sponsored groups.[26,41] For example, is the NPV of the "benign" *Afirma* test result on indeterminate nodules (based on cytologic-histologic correlation data at other independent institutions) sufficiently high to warrant the test result as clinically benign? How do the performance characteristics of the *Afirma* test for the AUS/FLUS diagnosis compare to that of a repeat thyroid FNA?[42] Could another type of ancillary study, such as immunohistochemistry, perform a similar function as a "rule-out" test?[43] How should the "suspicious" *Afirma* test result be interpreted and patients managed?

FUTURE TRENDS

More recently, the application of next-generation sequencing (NGS) technology has generated much interest in pathology.[44] This system is well suited for FNA cytology because only a small amount of tissue (10 ng of DNA) is required and the technology allows for the simultaneous sequencing of millions of short nucleic acid sequences in a parallel array. NGS has advantages over the more traditional techniques, such as Sanger sequencing, by sequencing large genomic regions and providing enhanced sensitivity in detecting genetic variants. For thyroid specimens, less common genetic alterations, such as mutations in *PIKCA, AKT1, PTEN,* and *p53* and gene rearrangements involving *BRAF* and *NTRK1* may be detected more effectively. Expanding the molecular panel through the use of NGS has the potential to improve its PPV as well as its NPV.[45] Comparable technologies may be adopted by commercial sources in improving their test accuracy. In time, the performance characteristics of the molecular panel and GEC tests may approach each other. As the technology matures, we can expect to have the combination of traditional thyroid cytology and molecular testing to provide a clearer view of the "indeterminate" cases.

REFERENCES

1. Ali SZ. Thyroid cytopathology: Bethesda and beyond. Acta Cytol 2011;55:4–12.
2. Nikiforov YE, Nikiforova MN. Molecular genetics and diagnosis of thyroid cancer. Nat Rev Endocrinol 2011;7:569–80.
3. Ohori NP, Schoedel KE. Thyroid cytology: challenges in the pursuit of low-grade malignancies. Radiol Clin North Am 2011;49:435–51.
4. Ohori NP, Schoedel KE. Variability in the atypia of undetermined significance/follicular lesion of undetermined significance diagnosis in the Bethesda system for reporting thyroid cytopathology: sources and recommendations. Acta Cytol 2011;55:492–8.
5. Knoepp SM, Roh MH. Ancillary techniques on direct-smear aspirate slides: a significant evolution for cytopathology techniques. Cancer Cytopathol 2013;121:120–8.
6. Fadda G, Rossi ED, Mulè A, et al. Diagnostic efficacy of immunocytochemistry on fine needle aspiration biopsies processed by thin-layer cytology. Acta Cytol 2006;50:129–35.
7. Rossi ED, Martini M, Capodimonti S, et al. Diagnostic and prognostic value of immunocytochemistry and BRAF mutation analysis on liquid-based biopsies of thyroid neoplasms suspicious for carcinoma. Eur J Endocrinol 2013;168:853–9.

8. Nga ME, Lim GS, Soh CH, et al. HBME-1 and CK19 are highly discriminatory in the cytological diagnosis of papillary thyroid carcinoma. Diagn Cytopathol 2008;36:550–6.

9. Saleh HA, Feng J, Tabassum F, et al. Differential expression of galectin-3, CK19, HBME1, and Ret oncoprotein in the diagnosis of thyroid neoplasms by fine needle aspiration biopsy. Cytojournal 2009;6:18.

10. Schmitt AC, Cohen C, Siddiqui MT. Paired box gene 8, HBME-1, and cytokeratin 19 expression in preoperative fine-needle aspiration of papillary thyroid carcinoma: diagnostic utility. Cancer Cytopathol 2010; 118:196–202.

11. Sack MJ, Astengo-Osuna C, Lin BT, et al. HBME-1 immunostaining in thyroid fine-needle aspirations: a useful marker in the diagnosis of carcinoma. Mod Pathol 1997;10:668–74.

12. Capper D, Preusser M, Habel A, et al. Assessment of BRAF V600E mutation status by immunohistochemistry with a mutation-specific monoclonal antibody. Acta Neuropathol 2011;122:11–9.

13. Bullock M, O'Neill C, Chou A, et al. Utilization of a MAB for BRAF(V600E) detection in papillary thyroid carcinoma. Endocr Relat Cancer 2012;19: 779–84.

14. Koperek O, Kornauth C, Capper D, et al. Immunohistochemical detection of the BRAF V600E-mutated protein in papillary thyroid carcinoma. Am J Surg Pathol 2012;36:844–50 [Erratum appears in Am J Surg Pathol 2012;36:1578].

15. Ghossein RA, Katabi N, Fagin JA. Immunohistochemical detection of mutated BRAF V600E supports the clonal origin of BRAF-induced thyroid cancers along the spectrum of disease progression. J Clin Endocrinol Metab 2013;98:E1414–21.

16. Nikiforov YE, Ohori NP, Hodak SP, et al. Impact of mutational testing on the diagnosis and management of patients with cytologically indeterminate thyroid nodules: a prospective analysis of 1056 FNA samples. J Clin Endocrinol Metab 2011;96: 3390–7.

17. Nikiforov YE, Steward DL, Robinson-Smith TM, et al. Molecular testing for mutations in improving the fine-needle aspiration diagnosis of thyroid nodules. J Clin Endocrinol Metab 2009;94:2092–8.

18. Cantara S, Capezzone M, Marchisotta S, et al. Impact of proto-oncogene mutation detection in cytological specimens from thyroid nodules improves the diagnostic accuracy of cytology. J Clin Endocrinol Metab 2010;95:1365–9.

19. Nikiforov YE. Molecular diagnostics of thyroid tumors. Arch Pathol Lab Med 2011;135:569–77.

20. Ohori NP, Singhal R, Nikiforova MN, et al. BRAF mutation detection in indeterminate thyroid cytology specimens: underlying cytologic, molecular, and pathologic characteristics of papillary thyroid carcinoma. Cancer Cytopathol 2013;121:197–205.

21. Pennelli G, Vianello F, Barollo S, et al. BRAF (K601E) mutation in a patient with a follicular thyroid carcinoma. Thyroid 2011;21(12):1393–6.

22. Soares P, Trovisco V, Rocha AS, et al. BRAF mutations and RET/PTC rearrangements are alternative events in the etiopathogenesis of PTC. Oncogene 2003;22:4578–80.

23. Gupta N, Dasyam AK, Carty SE, et al. RAS mutations in thyroid FNA specimens are highly predictive of predominantly low-risk follicular-pattern cancers. J Clin Endocrinol Metab 2013;98:E914–22.

24. Ohori NP, Nikiforova MN, Schoedel KE, et al. Contribution of molecular testing to thyroid fine-needle aspiration cytology of "follicular lesion of undetermined significance/atypia of undetermined significance". Cancer Cytopathol 2010;118:17–23.

25. Ohori NP, Wolfe J, Hodak SP, et al. "Colloid-rich" follicular neoplasm/suspicious for follicular neoplasm thyroid fine-needle aspiration specimens: cytologic, histologic, and molecular basis for considering an alternate view. Cancer Cytopathol 2013. http://dx.doi.org/10.1002/cncy.21333.

26. Nikiforov YE, Yip L, Nikiforova MN. New strategies in diagnosing cancer in thyroid nodules: impact of molecular markers. Clin Cancer Res 2013;19:2283–8.

27. Yip L, Farris C, Kabaker AS, et al. Cost impact of molecular testing for indeterminate thyroid nodule fine-needle aspiration biopsies. J Clin Endocrinol Metab 2012;97:1905–12.

28. Nikiforv YE, Ohori NP. Follicular carcinoma. In: Nikiforov YE, Biddinger PW, Thompson LD, editors. Diagnostic pathology and molecular genetics of the thyroid. 2nd edition. Philadelphia: Lippincott Williams & Wilkins; 2012. p. 152–82.

29. Zhu Z, Gandhi M, Nikiforova MN, et al. Molecular profile and clinico-pathologic features of the follicular variant of papillary thyroid carcinoma. An unusually high prevalence of ras mutations. Am J Clin Pathol 2003;120:71–7.

30. Fagin JA. Minireview: branded from the start-distinct oncogenic initiating events may determine tumor fate in the thyroid. Mol Endocrinol 2002;16: 903–11.

31. Burns JS, Blaydes JP, Wright PA, et al. Stepwise transformation of primary thyroid epithelial cells by mutant Ha-ras oncogene: an in vitro model of tumor progression. Mol Carcinog 1992;6:129–39.

32. Chudova D, Wilde JI, Wang ET, et al. Molecular classification of thyroid nodules using high-dimensionality genomic data. J Clin Endocrinol Metab 2010;95:5296–304.

33. Walsh PS, Wilde JI, Tom EY, et al. Analytical performance verification of a molecular diagnostic for cytology-indeterminate thyroid nodules. J Clin Endocrinol Metab 2012;97:E2297–306.

34. Alexander EK, Kennedy GC, Baloch ZW, et al. Preoperative diagnosis of benign thyroid nodules with

indeterminate cytology. N Engl J Med 2012;367: 705–15.

35. Ward LS, Kloos RT. Molecular markers in the diagnosis of thyroid nodules. Arq Bras Endocrinol Metabol 2013;57:89–97.

36. Duick DS, Klopper JP, Diggans JC, et al. The impact of benign gene expression classifier test results on the endocrinologist-patient decision to operate on patients with thyroid nodules with indeterminate fine-needle aspiration cytopathology. Thyroid 2012; 22:996–1001.

37. DeLellis RA, Lloyd RV, Heitz PU, et al, editors. World Health Organization classification of tumours. Pathology and genetics: tumours of endocrine organs. Lyon (France): IARC Press; 2004.

38. Elsheikh TM, Asa SL, Chan JK, et al. Interobserver and intraobserver variation among experts in the diagnosis of thyroid follicular lesions with borderline nuclear features of papillary carcinoma. Am J Clin Pathol 2008;130:736–44.

39. Li H, Robinson KA, Anton B, et al. Cost-effectiveness of a novel molecular test for cytologically indeterminate thyroid nodules. J Clin Endocrinol Metab 2011; 96:E1719–26.

40. Kloos RT, Reynolds JD, Walsh PS, et al. Does addition of BRAF V600E mutation testing modify sensitivity or specificity of the Afirma Gene Expression Classifier in cytologically indeterminate thyroid nodules? J Clin Endocrinol Metab 2013;98: E761–8.

41. Hodak SP, Rosenthal DS. Information for clinicians: commercially available molecular diagnosis testing in the evaluation of thyroid nodule fine-needle aspiration specimens. Thyroid 2013;23:131–4.

42. Faquin WC. Can a gene-expression classifier with high negative predictive value solve the indeterminate thyroid fine-needle aspiration dilemma? Cancer Cytopathol 2013;121:116–9.

43. Rossi ED, Larocca LM, Fadda G. Can a gene-expression classifier with high negative predictive value solve the indeterminate thyroid fine-needle aspiration dilemma? Cancer Cytopathol 2013;121: 403.

44. Hadd AG, Houghton J, Choudhary A, et al. Targeted, high-depth, next-generation sequencing of cancer genes in formalin-fixed, paraffin-embedded and fine-needle aspiration tumor specimens. J Mol Diagn 2013;15:234–47.

45. Nikiforova MN, Wald AI, Roy S, et al. Targeted next-generation sequencing panel (ThyroSeq) for detection of mutations in thyroid cancer. J Clin Endocrinol Metab 2013;98(11):E1852–60.

Cytology of the Salivary Glands

Raja R. Seethala, MD

KEYWORDS

• Salivary gland • Cytology • Immunohistochemistry • Molecular

ABSTRACT

Common usage of fine-needle aspirate (FNA) for salivary gland lesions is the preoperative determination of whether a lesion is neoplastic, its lineage, and if neoplastic, whether it is low grade/benign, or high grade. Immunohistochemical stains can be performed on cell blocks to determine lineage and help refine diagnosis, although their performance is not always equivalent to that seen in surgical specimens. Several characteristic translocations have been described in various entities in these categories, and these can be evaluated using fluorescence in situ hybridization. In the future, high-throughput next-generation sequencing panels may further refine cytologic diagnosis in salivary tumors.

INTRODUCTION

The main objective of fine-needle aspirate biopsy (FNAB) in salivary gland lesions is to provide an assessment of a salivary gland nodule that can influence the decision for surgical intervention, as well as extent of surgery. Here, priorities for the cytopathologist can be summarized as follows: (1) distinction between neoplastic and non-neoplastic lesions, (2) lineage determination for neoplasms (ie, epithelial, hematolymphoid, melanocytic, and mesenchymal tumor categories), and (3) separation of benign/low-grade tumors from high-grade tumors. For high-grade malignancies, separation of primary tumors from metastases is often a priority as well.[1–10] Specific diagnosis is actually not necessary for an informative FNAB, and may be challenging if not impossible in many cases, given the considerable cytologic overlap between various entities.[3,11,12]

The performance of FNAB in obtaining the objectives outlined previously relies mainly on a strong foundation in traditional morphologic assessment. But even in experienced hands, there are several pitfalls and deficiencies in cytologic evaluation. Thus, akin to surgical pathology, a role for immunohistochemical and even molecular studies on aspirate material has emerged to refine diagnosis. This article focuses mainly on the application of immunohistochemical and molecular testing as applied to the salivary epithelial neoplasms.

DIFFERENTIAL DIAGNOSIS

Salivary gland tumors are arguably the most diverse group of neoplasms per unit of total body volume.[13] This diversity, as well as morphologic overlap between several tumor types, make FNAB diagnosis very challenging. Proper diagnosis on surgical specimens requires adequate sampling and an algorithmic approach; the aforementioned diversity makes "wallpaper matching" potentially treacherous. FNAB diagnosis also benefits from an algorithmic approach, but without a unifying architectural configuration or "border" as seen on paraffin sections of a tumor resection, aspirates are paradoxically a more complex amalgamation of parameters.[1–10]

FNAB, as alluded to previously, also relies heavily on cellularity and stromal/extracellular characteristics. Because non-neoplastic considerations have not been preselected away from the differential diagnosis (surgical resections are more likely to be performed for tumors), these still

Department of Pathology, University of Pittsburgh Medical Center, A614.X PUH, 200 Lothrop Street, Pittsburgh, PA 15213, USA
E-mail address: seethalarr@upmc.edu

Surgical Pathology 7 (2014) 61–75
http://dx.doi.org/10.1016/j.path.2013.10.006

come into play and background inflammatory cell milieu thus becomes important. Furthermore, tinctorial qualities for a given tumor may vary on FNA smears in comparison with tissue sections, given the difference in stain preparation. For instance, as clear cell change is often composed of a combination of glycogenation, fixation, and staining, tumors that have clear-cell morphology on tissue sections may have a more oncocytoid appearance on aspirate material. Additionally, on FNA smears, cytoplasmic characteristics for myoepithelial and occasionally acinar cells may be stripped and absent altogether, imparting a basaloid appearance to a tumor that would be clear cell or oncocytic on histologic sections. Similar to histologic sections, cell constituents in a tumor are important on FNA, and here cell shape and size become even important for this determination.[1–10]

A detailed differential diagnostic approach is beyond the scope of this article. However, key FNAB categories that are encountered include the cellular/basaloid aspirate, the oncocytic or oncocytoid aspirate, cystic aspirate, and the lymphoid background rich aspirate. For this discussion, only epithelial neoplasms will be considered.

The cellular or basaloid aspirate commonly includes cellular pleomorphic adenoma, myoepithelioma, basal cell adenoma/adenocarcinoma, and adenoid cystic carcinoma (Table 1). Of these, adenoid cystic carcinoma is considerably more aggressive and is thus useful to recognize. All tumors in this category contain a mixture of ductal and myoepithelial cells, but certain characteristics, although often subtle, may be useful in separating these groups. Even cellular pleomorphic adenomas have areas containing the characteristic feathery myoxid matrix that appears metachromatic magenta on a Romanowsky-type stain (Fig. 1A, B). In contrast to the other categories, pleomorphic adenomas tend to have more cell heterogeneity, often containing plasmacytoid myoepithelial cells, ductal cells, and spindled stromal cells. Tumor cells that are embedded within the stroma may have a stellate or spindled appearance.[14,15] Myoepithelioma is not usually distinguishable from pleomorphic adenoma based on FNA alone given the considerable overlap, but the presence of ductal elements, if identified, would exclude this diagnosis.[16,17] Basal cell adenomas and basal cell adenocarcinomas are more uniform cytomorphologically (hence, the historic term monomorphic adenoma) and have a more collagenized stroma, although they still often have interdigitating tumor cells interspersed within (Fig. 2).[18–21] In contrast, adenoid cystic carcinoma is exceptionally monomorphic and contains angulated hyperchromatic nuclei with exceptionally scant cytoplasm with characteristic cylinders of matrix around which tumor cells are arranged, sharply demarcated rather than intermingling like the other categories (Fig. 3). One exception is the membranous variant of basal cell adenoma/adenocarcinoma, which has stroma that is very similar to that of adenoid cystic carcinoma.[18,22] But the nuclei of adenoid cystic carcinoma have coarser heterochromatin and a more irregularly shaped nucleolus than the other entities (see Fig. 3, inset).[23]

The oncocytic or oncocytoid aspirate has a broad differential diagnosis, but main considerations include oncocytoma, oncocytic cystadenoma, Warthin tumor, mucoepidermoid carcinoma, acinic cell carcinoma, mammary

---

Table 1
Key differential diagnostic considerations for the cellular basaloid aspirate

Diagnosis	Cytonuclear Features	Stromal/Background Characteristics
Pleomorphic adenoma	Diverse: bland ductal cells, plasmacytoid, epithelioid, and spindled cells	Myxoid with interspersed spindled to stellate cells Metachromatic on Romanowsky stain
Myoepithelioma	Bland plasmacytoid, epithelioid, and spindled cells, no ductal component	Myxoid to hyaline, less prominent than in pleomorphic adenoma
Basal cell adenoma/ Adenocarcinoma	Monomorphic ovoid cells with scant cytoplasm, can have ductal or squamous metaplasia, occasional peripheral palisading	Collagenized stroma with interdigitating tumor cells[a]
Adenoid cystic carcinoma	Monomorphic angulated hyperchromatic cells with angulated irregular nuclei	Cylinders of hyaline stroma with a peripheral arrangement tumor cells

[a] Membranous variant may have adenoid cystic like stroma.

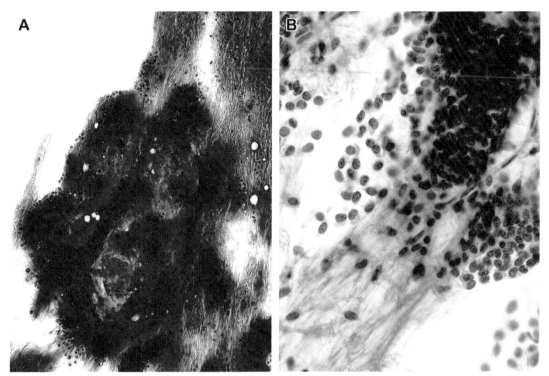

Fig. 1. Pleomorphic adenoma. (*A*) Classic low-power appearance of an aspirate of this tumor on a Romanowsky-based stain demonstrating the bright magenta fibrillary matrix particles (Diff Quick, original magnification ×100). (*B*) Even in more cellular examples, the tumor cells blend into this fibrillary stroma in a spindled or stellate fashion (Papanicoulou, original magnification ×400).

Fig. 2. Basal cell adenoma. This tumor consists of monomorphic basaloid cells embedded in a more hyaline or fibrous stroma than pleomorphic adenoma, although unlike adenoid cystic carcinoma, tumor cells still interdigitate with the stroma to a large extent (Papanicoulou, original magnification ×400).

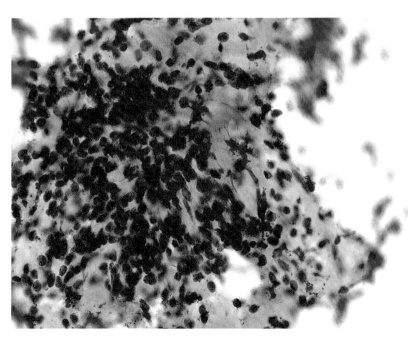

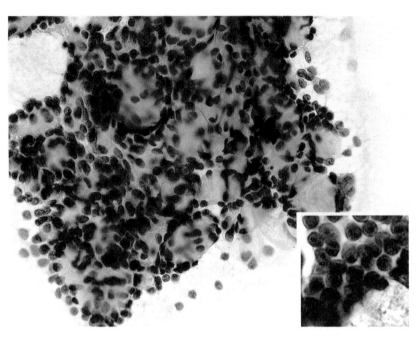

Fig. 3. Adenoid cystic carcinoma. This tumor is also basaloid, although tumor cells are angulated and characteristically arranged around hyaline cylinders, as seen here (Papanicoulou, original magnification ×400). Inset: Adenoid cystic carcinoma tends to have coarser chromatin and more irregular nucleoli than other tumors in the differential diagnosis (Papanicoulou, original magnification x600).

analogue secretory carcinoma, and salivary duct carcinoma (**Table 2**). Oncocytoma, oncocytic cystadenoma, and Warthin tumor have a similar cytomorphologic appearance in that aspirates contain tumor cells with abundant granular eosinophilic (or cyanophilic to orangeophilic on Papanicoulou stain) cytoplasm and small round indistinct nuclei. Distinction is based on a cyst fluid background that is absent in oncocytoma, and a lymphoid background, which defines Warthin tumor (**Fig. 4**).[24–26] Mucoepidermoid carcinoma often shows a prominent oncocytic

Table 2
Key differential diagnostic considerations for the oncocytic/oncocytoid, cystic and lymphoid rich aspirate

Diagnosis	Cytonuclear Features	Stromal/Background Characteristics
Warthin tumor/ Oncocytoma/Oncocytic cystadenoma	Abundant granular cytoplasm with bland indistinct nuclei.	Cyst content background in cystadenoma Cyst content and lymphoid background in Warthin tumor
Mucoepidermoid carcinoma	Mixture of mucous, epidermoid and basaloid intermediate-type cells, oncocytic cells may be prominent. Proportion and cytonuclear atypia varies with grade.	Mucoid or cyst content background Lymphoid background in a subset
Acinic cell carcinoma	Granular to vacuolated cytoplasm with basophilic zymogen granules, may have a prominent oncocytoid zymogen poor cell population.	May show cyst or lymphoid content background
Mammary analogue secretory carcinoma	Granular eosinophilic and frequently heavily vacuolated.	May show cyst or lymphoid content background
Salivary duct carcinoma	Pleomorphic granular to vacuolated oncocytoid cells. Nuclei often show prominent nucleoli.	Necrotic background and neutrophils not uncommon

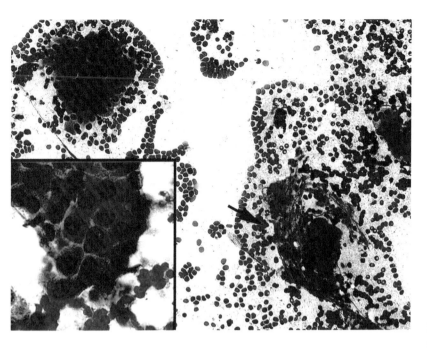

Fig. 4. Warthin tumor. This tumor consists of clusters of cells with abundant granular cytoplasm and bland nuclei. There is some granular debris in the background suggestive of cyst contents. Lymphoid tangles (*arrow*) are not uncommon (Diff-Quick, original magnification ×200). Inset: On Papanicoulou stain, the oncocytes may show a granular orange-ophilic cytoplasm with cyanophilic undertones, as seen here. Nuclei are small and monomorphic, although nucleoli may be visible (Papanicoulou, original magnification ×400).

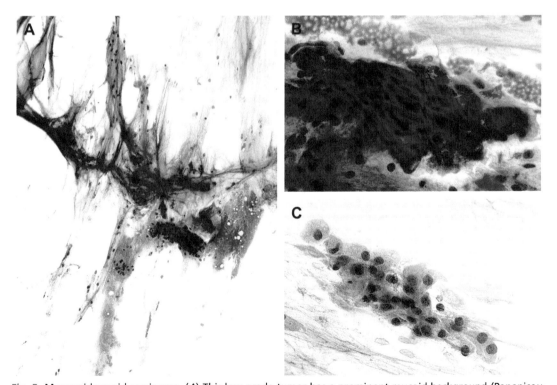

Fig. 5. Mucoepidermoid carcinoma. (*A*) This low-grade tumor has a prominent mucoid background (Papanicoulou, original magnification ×100). (*B*) Although cells tend to be polygonal with moderate amounts of granular cytoplasm, focal epidermoid differentiation is noted, as suggested by the orangeophilic streaming of nuclei in this cell cluster (Papanicoulou, original magnification ×400). (*C*) Mucocytes are polygonal and vacuolated and may resemble muciphages (Papanicoulou, original magnification ×400).

component, lymphoid stroma, and may be solid or cystic depending on grade, but should show a mixture of epidermoid and mucous cells as well (**Fig. 5A–C**).[27,28] One caveat is that an "infarcted" Warthin tumor may show squamous and mucous cell metaplasia, making distinction very difficult on FNAB. Classic acinic cell carcinoma is zymogen granule rich and has a more basophilic cytoplasm, but occasionally overlaps with oncocytic lesions. Recognition of the more classic areas is important to the diagnosis here (**Fig. 6A**).[29] The recently described mammary analogue secretory carcinoma and salivary duct carcinoma also are composed of tumor cells that have an oncocytoid appearance with abundant granular cytoplasm. However, mammary analogue secretory carcinoma is quite mucin rich and shows a heavily vacuolated cytoplasm (see **Fig. 6B**).[30] Salivary duct carcinoma can be distinguished in that it is prototypically high grade and will show considerable cytonuclear pleomorphism with prominent nucleoli (**Fig. 7**). Tumor necrosis is not uncommon.[31,32]

Interestingly, many of the oncocytic lesions noted previously comprise the differential diagnosis for cystic and lymphoid background-rich aspirates, because, in addition to Warthin tumor, mucoepidermoid carcinoma, acinic cell carcinoma, and mammary analogue secretory carcinoma may be both cystic and have a rich lymphoid stroma. On FNAB, the differential for lymphoid-rich and cystic lesions may also include non-neoplastic entities, including sialadenitis, sialocyst, and lymphoepithelial cyst. Here, clinical appearance (discrete mass vs diffuse enlargement) is useful. Additionally, non-neoplastic aspirates often contain fewer epithelial elements.

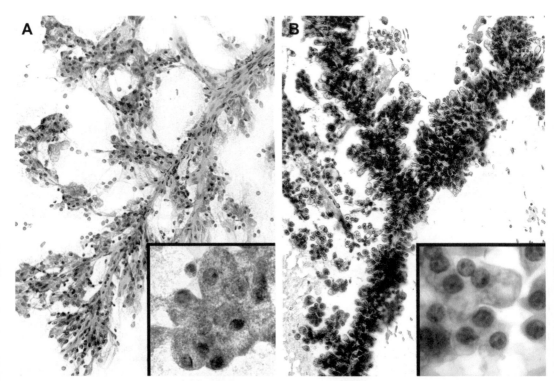

Fig. 6. Acinic cell carcinoma and mammary analogue secretory carcinoma. (*A*) Acinic cell carcinoma may show an arborizing papillary architecture on FNAB (Papanicoulou, original magnification ×100). Inset: The tumor cells are fairly bland and demonstrate numerous zymogen granules (Papanicoulou, original magnification ×400). (*B*) Mammary analogue secretory carcinoma can essentially recapitulate any pattern seen in acinic cell carcinoma on FNAB (Papanicoulou, original magnification ×100). Inset: The main distinction cytomorphologically is the extent of vacuolization typical of mammary analogue secretory carcinoma (Papanicoulou, original magnification ×400).

Fig. 7. Salivary duct carcinoma. Akin to other oncocytoid aspirates, the tumor cells contain abundant granular to vacuolated cytoplasm, but here there is profound nuclear pleomorphism, even at this magnification, and there is a background of neutrophils and debris (Diff Quick, original magnification ×200). Inset: On higher magnification, nuclear size and shape variation is marked, and tumor cells show very prominent enlarged eosinophilic nucleoli (Papanicoulou, original magnification ×400).

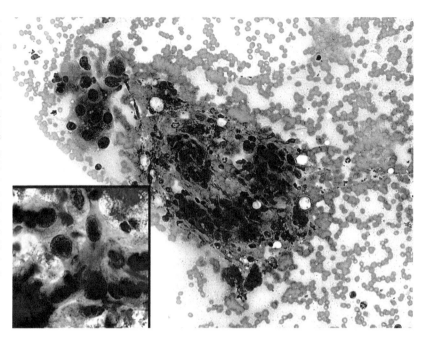

ANCILLARY STUDIES

SPECIAL STAINS

Histochemical stains are often used to highlight stromal or cytoplasmic components. For instance, Mucicarmine, periodic acid-Schiff (PAS) after diastase treatment, and Alcian blue (pH 2.5) stains all can highlight intracytoplasmic and luminal mucin, which are important to a variety of tumor types, most notably mucoepidermoid carcinoma. PAS after diastase also highlights zymogen granules in acinic cell carcinoma. Phosphotungstic acid hematoxylin stain highlights the mitochondria in oncocytes, and on frozen tissue, Oil Red O remains one of the best methods to confirm sebaceous differentiation by highlighting lipid droplets.

IMMUNOHISTOCHEMISTRY

Immunohistochemical stains have evolved into increasingly more useful adjuncts to morphologic assessment. They are useful in delineating epithelial tumors from lymphoma, sarcoma, and melanoma. Additionally, available immunohistochemical stains can help in accurate classification of different salivary tumor types. However, effective utilization of immunostains requires interpretation in the context of morphologic features (ie, cell compartments that are positive, intensity, distribution). Staining interpretation should be applied cautiously, particularly in the case of FNAB. The broad utility of immunostains is in the

determination of cell types within the tumor: ductal (epithelial), myoepithelial, basal, or acinar (Table 3). As a rule, lower molecular weight keratins are more strongly expressed in ductal-type tumors, whereas higher molecular weight keratins and p63 are expressed in the basal, myoepithelial, or squamous components of tumors.[33–36] Myoepithelial cells additionally express vimentin and muscle markers (actin, calponin) to varying degrees.[37–39] S100, although regarded as a myoepithelial marker, is often expressed in ductal-type tumors, such as canalicular adenoma and polymorphous low-grade adenocarcinoma.[36] Recently, DOG1 and SOX10 have been shown to favor an acinar phenotype (see Table 3).[40,41] Additionally, certain markers, such as androgen receptor, GCDFP15 (in salivary duct carcinoma),[42] and c-Kit (in adenoid cystic carcinoma)[43] are preferentially expressed in certain tumor types.

MOLECULAR TESTING

Molecular testing is now feasible both on cell blocks and aspirate material. Several frequent (and occasionally defining) translocations, amplifications, and mutations that can be assessed using fluorescence in situ hybridization (FISH)-based or polymerase chain reaction (PCR)-based methods have been described (Table 4). Defining translocations include the t(12;22)(q13;p12) translocation resulting in the *EWSR1-ATF1* fusion seen in hyalinizing clear cell carcinoma[44] and the

Table 3
Basic immunohistochemical staining properties and cell components

	Basal Cells	Myoepithelial Cells	Ductal Cells	Acinar Cells
Distribution within ductoacinar units	Throughout; more prominent in larger ducts	Acini and intercalated ducts	Throughout	Acini
Localization with respect to lumen	Abluminal; stratified in larger ducts	Abluminal	Luminal	Luminal
Low molecular weight cytokeratins (CAM 5.2, CK7, CK19)	Weak to negative	Weak to negative (variable in tumors)	Strongly positive	Variable
High molecular weight cytokeratins (CK 5/6, 34βE12)	Strongly positive	Strongly positive (variable in tumors)	Variable (more likely to be positive in larger ducts)	Negative
p63	Positive	Positive	Negative	Negative
Muscle markers (actin, calponin, smooth muscle myosin heavy chain)	Negative	Positive	Negative	Negative
DOG-1, SOX-10	Negative	Negative	Focal in intercalated ducts; otherwise negative	Positive, serous more than mucous

Table 4
Common known molecular alterations in primary salivary gland tumors

Tumor	Chromosomal Alteration	Gene	Prevalence (%)
Pleomorphic adenoma	8q12	*PLAG1*	25–30
	12q13–15 Rearrangements	*HMGA2*	10–15
Membranous basal cell adenoma/Adenocarcinoma	16q12–13 Loss of heterozygosity/mutation	*CYLD1*	75–80
Mucoepidermoid carcinoma	t(11;19)(q21;p13)	*CRTC1-MAML2*	40–80
	t(11;15)(q21;q26)	*CRTC3-MAML2*	~5
Salivary duct carcinoma	17q21.1 Amplification	*ERBB2*	~40
Adenoid cystic carcinoma	t(6;9)(q22–23;p23–24)	*MYB-NFIB*	25–50
Mammary analogue secretory carcinoma	t(12;15)(p13;q25)	*ETV6-NRTK3*	~100 (defining)
Hyalinizing clear cell carcinoma	t(12;22)(q21;q12)	*EWSR1-ATF1*	~80–90 (defining)

t(12;15)(p13;q25) translocation resulting in the *ETV6-NTRK3* fusion seen in mammary analogue secretory carcinoma,[45] and can establish these diagnoses even on FNAB. Furthermore, the vast majority of mucoepidermoid carcinomas harbor a *CRTC1* or *CRTC3-MAML2* fusion (t[11;19][q21–22;p13][46] or t[11;15][q21;q26][47] translocations, respectively), and, thus, identification of one of these translocations is diagnostic. Chiosea and colleagues,[48] based on prospective in-house clinical experience, have documented the feasibility of this test on aspirate material. Recently, the t(6;9)(q22–23;p23–24) translocation that results in a *MYB-NFIB* fusion has been described in adenoid cystic carcinoma. Although the prevalence of this translocation varies between 25% and 100%,[49] positive translocation status is specific for adenoid cystic carcinoma and can thus have utility.

THERAPEUTIC AND PROGNOSTIC APPLICATIONS

Although by refining diagnosis on FNAB, ancillary testing influences therapeutic modalities pursued, direct therapeutic applications of such studies are of limited utility, especially on FNAB, as the vast majority of tumors are treated initially, and often definitively, with surgical approach. Additionally, certain markers that are therapeutic targets for other organ sites do not appear effective in predicting response in salivary carcinomas. For instance, although c-Kit is ubiquitously expressed in adenoid cystic carcinoma, the few studies available have shown partial or no response to imatinib,[50] which targets this receptor. However, recent identification of activating FGFR-2 mutations in a subset of tumors establish another

potential target.[51] Attempts at demonstrating response in salivary duct carcinoma to transtuzimab, which targets Her-2/Neu have yielded some favorable results but mainly on a small scale.[52] Recently, however, few cases in which antiandrogen therapy in this tumor type have resulted in favorable response have been described.[53,54] Also, PIK3CA mutations now potentially offer new therapeutic targets for salivary duct carcinoma as well.[55]

Perhaps the main prognostic utility of ancillary testing is with respect to the *CRTC1* or *CRTC3-MAML2* translocations seen in mucoepidermoid carcinoma. Overall, translocation positivity has been noted to correlate with a lower grade and better prognosis, but the strength of this prognostic indicator independent of stage and accurate categorization of high-grade tumors is debated in the literature.[56] Of note, p16 deletions have been noted in limited series to negate the favorable prognosis of positive translocation status, mainly in high-grade mucoepidermoid carcinoma.[57]

PRACTICAL APPLICATIONS

The feasibility of ancillary testing depends on methodology, as well as quality of aspirate material. However, immunohistochemistry and FISH are quite readily performed. With the existence of cell block material, the immunohistochemical armamentarium for FNA is essentially equivalent to that of surgical specimens. The application of ancillary studies has yielded mixed results, however, from a practical perspective (see Pitfalls).

For example, the cellular basaloid salivary aspirate poses a significant challenge for appropriate categorization given the paucity of stromal elements, and the inclusion of adenoid cystic carcinoma, which has a distinct management in comparison with the other considerations, in the differential diagnosis. As with surgical specimens, adenoid cystic carcinomas typically express c-kit (**Fig. 8**) on FNAB. However, this marker actually does not perform as well on FNA in discriminating between mimics, even with different antibodies.[58] But taking a different approach, glial fibrillary acidic protein and CD57 positivity successfully distinguishes pleomorphic adenoma from other considerations, notably adenoid cystic carcinoma, although not entirely sensitive for this diagnosis. Another caveat is that other basaloid entities are not excluded by GFAP, CD57 negativity.[59]

The oncocytic or oncocytoid aspirate can be similarly challenging, whether cystic or solid, or with prominent lymphoid stroma. The low-grade differential diagnosis encompasses benign tumors and non-neoplastic lesions, such as Warthin tumor, oncocytic cystadenoma/salivary cyst, and low-grade malignancies, such as mucoepidermoid carcinoma, mammary analogue secretory carcinoma, and acinic cell carcinoma. To this end, FISH has tremendous potential utility

because it can definitively diagnose mucoepidermoid carcinoma and mammary analogue secretory carcinoma. Griffith and colleagues[30] successfully applied this technique on cell block material to validate FISH testing for the *ETV6-NTRK3* translocation for mammary analogue secretory carcinoma on aspirate cell blocks and even describe a prospectively diagnosed case preceding surgical resection (**Fig. 9**A, C). Mammary analogue secretory carcinoma is also noted to be S100 and mammaglobin positive even on aspirate material (see **Fig. 9**B), although occasionally either or even both of these markers may be negative on an aspirate.[30] Chiosea and colleagues[48] also demonstrated that FNA material is adequate for testing for the *CRTC1/3-MAML* translocations in mucoepidermoid carcinoma. Given that up to 30% of mucoepidermoid carcinomas are negative for a known translocation, it must be noted, however, that a negative FISH result does not exclude this diagnosis. On the high-grade end of the oncocytoid spectrum, high-grade mucoepidermoid carcinoma, salivary duct carcinoma, and metastases enter the differential diagnosis. Although a subset of even

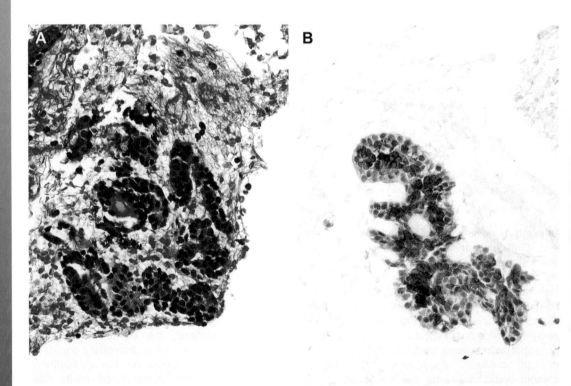

Fig. 8. c-kit immunohistochemistry in adenoid cystic carcinoma. (*A*) This cell block shows a few crushed bilayered tubules composed of intensely hyperchromatic nuclei (hematoxylin and eosin [H&E], original magnification ×400). (*B*) A c-kit immunostain is positive with a ductal accentuation (3,3'-Diaminobenzidine [DAB], original magnification ×400). However, this marker is not very specific on FNAB and should be used with caution.

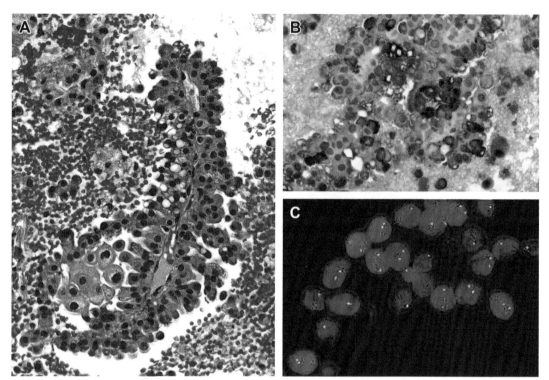

Fig. 9. Ancillary testing applied to mammary analogue secretory carcinoma. (*A*) Cell block showing a papillary growth and tumor cells that are unusually pleomorphic for this diagnosis containing granular and vacuolated cytoplasm, concerning perhaps for a more aggressive tumor, such as salivary duct carcinoma (H&E, original magnification ×400). (*B*) Mammaglobin is positive (DAB, original magnification ×400). (*C*) But FISH here for *ETV6* shows one intact yellow signal and one split red-green signal in almost all tumor cells consistent with a translocation thus confirming the diagnosis.

high-grade mucoepidermoid carcinomas harbor a *CRTC-MAML* translocation, negativity again does not exclude this diagnosis. Salivary duct carcinoma can be successfully established using androgen receptor immunohistochemistry (Fig. 10).[60] One caveat is that the cytonuclear features must be those of an intermediate to high-grade oncocytoid malignant neoplasm, because even pleomorphic adenomas with apocrine change may express these markers.[61]

Pitfalls
IN THE INTERPRETATION OF ANCILLARY TESTING ON FNA MATERIAL

! While a cell block allows virtually any immunohistochemical available for surgical specimens to be performed on FNA material, performance of markers (ie, c-kit selectivity for adenoid cystic carcinoma) may not be as strong in comparison with surgical material.

! Some immunohistochemical markers (ie, S100 and mammaglobin in mammary analogue secretory carcinoma) may only be focally expressed and thus may appear negative on FNA material, given its limited nature.

! Immunoreactivity must always be considered only in the context of the cytonuclear features, as certain markers (ie, androgen receptor) may be expressed in a variety of tumor types and should thus not be the sole reason to establish a diagnosis (in this example, salivary duct carcinoma).

! Determining translocation status in a tumor may be useful to confirm a specific diagnosis on FNA, but negativity for a certain translocations (ie, CRTC1/3-MAML) do not necessarily exclude the diagnosis in consideration (in this example, mucoepidermoid carcinoma)

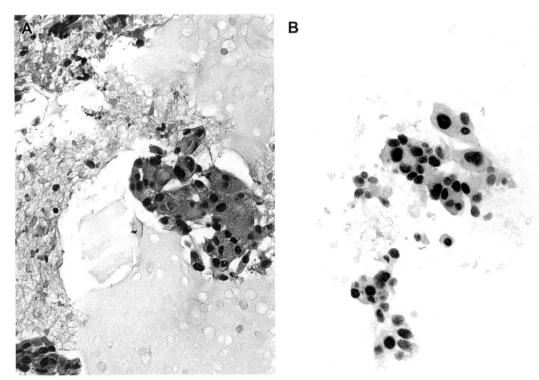

Fig. 10. Androgen receptor confirming salivary duct carcinoma. (*A*) Cell block demonstrates a pleomorphic tumor with granular and vacuolated eosinophilic cytoplasm (H&E, original magnification ×400). (*B*) Androgen receptor is strongly positive (DAB, original magnification ×400).

FUTURE TRENDS

For better or worse, the need to "do more with less" will be the norm in medicine in the near future. As such, FNA material will be increasingly used as the substrate for ancillary testing. As molecular techniques become increasingly feasible, even PCR-based modalities will be incorporated into the approach to salivary gland tumors. Thyroid FNA experience can serve as the template for such advances in salivary tumors. It is now well established that placing one FNA pass directly into nucleic acid fixative yields adequate DNA and even RNA for subsequent molecular testing in thyroid FNA.[62] Ultimately, as the molecular understanding of salivary tumors increases, a high-throughput panel-based molecular assay will likely be beneficial in stratifying lesions. Next-generation sequencing panels fulfilling this purpose are already being incorporated for thyroid FNA and will likely find their way to salivary FNA as well.[63]

Specific markers not yet currently tested but on the horizon for both immunohistochemical and molecular assays may further refine the basaloid branch of the diagnostic tree and include PLAG1 and HMGA2 immunohistochemistry and FISH for pleomorphic adenoma, nuclear beta catenin immunohistochemistry for basal cell adenoma, and MYB immunohistochemistry and FISH for adenoid cystic carcinoma. Recently, yet another *EWSR1* translocation (with *POU5F1*) has been described in association with high-grade mucoepidermoid carcinoma.[64]

Thus, in summary, the histologic diversity of salivary gland neoplasms pose tremendous obstacles for the appropriate classification on FNA. However, with the increasing feasibility of immunohistochemistry, FISH, and even PCR-based testing on FNA material, the morphologic classification can be further refined. As with other organ sites, a panel-based high-throughput approach with next-generation sequencing techniques will be increasingly used on salivary FNA for diagnostic and perhaps therapeutic purposes.

REFERENCES

1. O'Dwyer P, Farrar WB, James AG, et al. Needle aspiration biopsy of major salivary gland tumors. Its value. Cancer 1986;57(3):554–7.
2. Cohen MB, Ljung BM, Boles R. Salivary gland tumors. Fine-needle aspiration vs frozen-section diagnosis. Arch Otolaryngol Head Neck Surg 1986;112(8):867–9.

3. Layfield LJ, Tan P, Glasgow BJ. Fine-needle aspiration of salivary gland lesions. Comparison with frozen sections and histologic findings. Arch Pathol Lab Med 1987;111(4):346–53.

4. Costas A, Castro P, Martin-Granizo R, et al. Fine needle aspiration biopsy (FNAB) for lesions of the salivary glands. Br J Oral Maxillofac Surg 2000; 38(5):539–42.

5. Wong DS, Li GK. The role of fine-needle aspiration cytology in the management of parotid tumors: a critical clinical appraisal. Head Neck 2000;22(5): 469–73.

6. Al-Khafaji BM, Nestok BR, Katz RL. Fine-needle aspiration of 154 parotid masses with histologic correlation: ten-year experience at the University of Texas M. D. Anderson Cancer Center. Cancer 1998;84(3):153–9.

7. Stewart CJ, MacKenzie K, McGarry GW, et al. Fine-needle aspiration cytology of salivary gland: a review of 341 cases. Diagn Cytopathol 2000;22(3):139–46.

8. Stanley MW. Selected problems in fine needle aspiration of head and neck masses. Mod Pathol 2002; 15(3):342–50.

9. Stanley MW, Lowhagen T. Fine needle aspiration of palpable masses. (MA): Butterworth-Heinnemann Oxford; 1993.

10. Que Hee CG. Fine needle aspiration cytology of parotid tumours: is it useful? ANZ J Surg 2001; 71(6):345–8.

11. Hughes JH, Volk EE, Wilbur DC, Cytopathology Resource Committee CoAP. Pitfalls in salivary gland fine-needle aspiration cytology: lessons from the College of American Pathologists Interlaboratory Comparison Program in Nongynecologic Cytology. Arch Pathol Lab Med 2005;129(1):26–31.

12. Layfield LJ, Glasgow BJ. Diagnosis of salivary gland tumors by fine-needle aspiration cytology: a review of clinical utility and pitfalls. Diagn Cytopathol 1991;7(3):267–72.

13. Eveson JW, Auclair PL, Gnepp DR, et al. Tumors of the salivary glands: introduction. In: Barnes EL, Eveson JW, Reichart P, et al, editors. World Health Organization classification of tumours: pathology & genetics. Head and Neck Tumours. Lyon (France): IARCPress; 2005. p. 221–2.

14. Kuwabara H, Kohno K, Kishida F, et al. Fine needle aspiration cytology of predominant plasmacytoid myoepithelial cells in pleomorphic adenoma of the palate. Acta Cytol 1997;41(5):1637–40.

15. Viguer JM, Vicandi B, Jimenez-Heffernan JA, et al. Fine needle aspiration cytology of pleomorphic adenoma. An analysis of 212 cases. Acta Cytol 1997;41(3):786–94.

16. Dodd LG, Caraway NP, Luna MA, et al. Myoepithelioma of the parotid. Report of a case initially examined by fine needle aspiration biopsy. Acta Cytol 1994;38(3):417–21.

17. Lopez JI, Ugalde A, Arostegui J, et al. Plasmacytoid myoepithelioma of the soft palate. Report of a case with cytologic, immunohistochemical and electron microscopic studies. Acta Cytol 2000; 44(4):647–52.

18. Stanley MW, Horwitz CA, Rollins SD, et al. Basal cell (monomorphic) and minimally pleomorphic adenomas of the salivary glands. Distinction from the solid (anaplastic) type of adenoid cystic carcinoma in fine-needle aspiration. Am J Clin Pathol 1996; 106(1):35–41.

19. Lopez JI, Ballestin C. Fine-needle aspiration cytology of a membranous basal cell adenoma arising in an intraparotid lymph node. Diagn Cytopathol 1993;9(6):668–72.

20. Sahu K, Pai RR, Pai KP. Basal cell adenoma, solid variant, diagnosed by fine needle aspiration cytology. Acta Cytol 1999;43(6):1198–200.

21. Galed-Placed I, Yebra-Pimentel MT. Synchronous, double parotid tumor: fine needle aspiration cytology diagnosis of the membranous basal cell adenoma component. Acta Cytol 2000;44(6): 1120–2.

22. Hajdu SI, Melamed MR. Limitations of aspiration cytology in the diagnosis of primary neoplasms. Acta Cytol 1984;28(3):337–45.

23. Yang GC, Waisman J. Distinguishing adenoid cystic carcinoma from cylindromatous adenomas in salivary fine-needle aspirates: the cytologic clues and their ultrastructural basis. Diagn Cytopathol 2006;34(4):284–8.

24. Zhang S, Bao R, Abreo F. Papillary oncocytic cystadenoma of the parotid glands: a report of 2 cases with varied cytologic features. Acta Cytol 2009; 53(4):445–8.

25. Layfield LJ, Gopez EV. Cystic lesions of the salivary glands: cytologic features in fine-needle aspiration biopsies. Diagn Cytopathol 2002;27(4):197–204.

26. Verma K, Kapila K. Salivary gland tumors with a prominent oncocytic component. Cytologic findings and differential diagnosis of oncocytomas and Warthin's tumor on fine needle aspirates. Acta Cytol 2003;47(2):221–6.

27. Klijanienko J, Vielh P. Fine-needle sampling of salivary gland lesions. IV. Review of 50 cases of mucoepidermoid carcinoma with histologic correlation. Diagn Cytopathol 1997;17(2):92–8.

28. Wade TV, Livolsi VA, Montone KT, et al. A cytohistologic correlation of mucoepidermoid carcinoma: emphasizing the rare oncocytic variant. Patholog Res Int 2011;2011:135796.

29. Klijanienko J, Vielh P. Fine-needle sample of salivary gland lesions. V: cytology of 22 cases of acinic cell carcinoma with histologic correlation. Diagn Cytopathol 1997;17(5):347–52.

30. Griffith CC, Stelow EB, Saqi A, et al. The cytological features of mammary analogue secretory

carcinoma: a series of 6 molecularly confirmed cases. Cancer Cytopathol 2013;121(5):234–41.

31. Gilcrease MZ, Guzman-Paz M, Froberg K, et al. Salivary duct carcinoma. Is a specific diagnosis possible by fine needle aspiration cytology? Acta Cytol 1998;42(6):1389–96.

32. Khurana KK, Pitman MB, Powers CN, et al. Diagnostic pitfalls of aspiration cytology of salivary duct carcinoma. Cancer 1997;81(6):373–8.

33. Reis-Filho JS, Schmitt FC. Taking advantage of basic research: p63 is a reliable myoepithelial and stem cell marker. Adv Anat Pathol 2002;9(5):280–9.

34. Seethala RR, LiVolsi VA, Zhang PJ, et al. Comparison of p63 and p73 expression in benign and malignant salivary gland lesions. Head Neck 2005;27(8):696–702.

35. Weber A, Langhanki L, Schutz A, et al. Expression profiles of p53, p63, and p73 in benign salivary gland tumors. Virchows Arch 2002;441(5):428–36.

36. Seethala RR, Barnes EL, Hunt JL. Epithelial-myoepithelial carcinoma: a review of the clinicopathologic spectrum and immunophenotypic characteristics in 61 tumors of the salivary glands and upper aerodigestive tract. Am J Surg Pathol 2007;31(1):44–57.

37. Alos L, Cardesa A, Bombi JA, et al. Myoepithelial tumors of salivary glands: a clinicopathologic, immunohistochemical, ultrastructural, and flowcytometric study. Semin Diagn Pathol 1996;13(2):138–47.

38. Takai Y, Dardick I, Mackay A, et al. Diagnostic criteria for neoplastic myoepithelial cells in pleomorphic adenomas and myoepitheliomas. Immunocytochemical detection of muscle-specific actin, cytokeratin 14, vimentin, and glial fibrillary acidic protein. Oral Surg Oral Med Oral Pathol Oral Radiol Endod 1995;79(3):330–41.

39. Furuse C, Sousa SO, Nunes FD, et al. Myoepithelial cell markers in salivary gland neoplasms. Int J Surg Pathol 2005;13(1):57–65.

40. Ohtomo R, Mori T, Shibata S, et al. SOX10 is a novel marker of acinus and intercalated duct differentiation in salivary gland tumors: a clue to the histogenesis for tumor diagnosis. Mod Pathol 2013;26(8):1041–50.

41. Chenevert J, Duvvuri U, Chiosea S, et al. DOG1: a novel marker of salivary acinar and intercalated duct differentiation. Mod Pathol 2012;25(7):919–29.

42. Fan CY, Wang J, Barnes EL. Expression of androgen receptor and prostatic specific markers in salivary duct carcinoma: an immunohistochemical analysis of 13 cases and review of the literature. Am J Surg Pathol 2000;24(4):579–86.

43. Penner CR, Folpe AL, Budnick SD. C-kit expression distinguishes salivary gland adenoid cystic carcinoma from polymorphous low-grade adenocarcinoma. Mod Pathol 2002;15(7):687–91.

44. Antonescu CR, Katabi N, Zhang L, et al. EWSR1-ATF1 fusion is a novel and consistent finding in hyalinizing clear-cell carcinoma of salivary gland. Genes Chromosomes Cancer 2011;50(7):559–70.

45. Skalova A, Vanecek T, Sima R, et al. Mammary analogue secretory carcinoma of salivary glands, containing the ETV6-NTRK3 fusion gene: a hitherto undescribed salivary gland tumor entity. Am J Surg Pathol 2010;34(5):599–608.

46. Tonon G, Modi S, Wu L, et al. t(11;19)(q21;p13) translocation in mucoepidermoid carcinoma creates a novel fusion product that disrupts a Notch signaling pathway. Nat Genet 2003;33(2):208–13.

47. Fehr A, Roser K, Heidorn K, et al. A new type of MAML2 fusion in mucoepidermoid carcinoma. Genes Chromosomes Cancer 2008;47(3):203–6.

48. Chiosea SI, Dacic S, Nikiforova MN, et al. Prospective testing of mucoepidermoid carcinoma for the MAML2 translocation: clinical implications. Laryngoscope 2012;122(8):1690–4.

49. Bell D, Hanna EY. Head and neck adenoid cystic carcinoma: what is new in biological markers and treatment? Curr Opin Otolaryngol Head Neck Surg 2013;21(2):124–9.

50. Pfeffer MR, Talmi Y, Catane R, et al. A phase II study of Imatinib for advanced adenoid cystic carcinoma of head and neck salivary glands. Oral Oncol 2007;43(1):33–6.

51. Stephens PJ, Davies HR, Mitani Y, et al. Whole exome sequencing of adenoid cystic carcinoma. J Clin Invest 2013;123(7):2965–8.

52. Limaye SA, Posner MR, Krane JF, et al. Trastuzumab for the treatment of salivary duct carcinoma. Oncologist 2013;18(3):294–300.

53. Jaspers HC, Verbist BM, Schoffelen R, et al. Androgen receptor-positive salivary duct carcinoma: a disease entity with promising new treatment options. J Clin Oncol 2011;29(16):e473–6.

54. Kuroda H, Sakurai T, Yamada M, et al. Effective treatment by both anti-androgen therapy and chemotherapy for a patient with advanced salivary duct carcinoma. Gan To Kagaku Ryoho 2011;38(4):627–30 [in Japanese].

55. Griffith CC, Seethala RR, Luvison A, et al. PIK3CA mutations and PTEN loss in salivary duct carcinomas. Am J Surg Pathol 2013;37(8):1201–7.

56. Seethala RR, Dacic S, Cieply K, et al. A reappraisal of the MECT1/MAML2 translocation in salivary mucoepidermoid carcinomas. Am J Surg Pathol 2010;34(8):1106–21.

57. Anzick SL, Chen WD, Park Y, et al. Unfavorable prognosis of CRTC1-MAML2 positive mucoepidermoid tumors with CDKN2A deletions. Genes Chromosomes Cancer 2010;49(1):59–69.

58. Chandan VS, Wilbur D, Faquin WC, et al. Is c-kit (CD117) immunolocalization in cell block preparations useful in the differentiation of adenoid cystic carcinoma from pleomorphic adenoma? Cancer 2004;102(4):207–9.
59. Shah SS, Chandan VS, Wilbur DC, et al. Glial fibrillary acidic protein and CD57 immunolocalization in cell block preparations is a useful adjunct in the diagnosis of pleomorphic adenoma. Arch Pathol Lab Med 2007;131(9):1373–7.
60. Moriki T, Ueta S, Takahashi T, et al. Salivary duct carcinoma: cytologic characteristics and application of androgen receptor immunostaining for diagnosis. Cancer 2001;93(5):344–50.
61. DeRoche TC, Hoschar AP, Hunt JL. Immunohistochemical evaluation of androgen receptor, HER-2/neu, and p53 in benign pleomorphic adenomas. Arch Pathol Lab Med 2008;132(12):1907–11.
62. Nikiforov YE. Molecular analysis of thyroid tumors. Mod Pathol 2011;24(Suppl 2):S34–43.
63. Nikiforova MN, Wald AI, Roy S, et al. Targeted next-generation sequencing panel (ThyroSeq) for detection of mutations in thyroid cancer. J Clin Endocrinol Metab 2013;98(11):E1852–60 [Epub ahead of print].
64. Stenman G. Fusion oncogenes in salivary gland tumors: molecular and clinical consequences. Head Neck Pathol 2013;7(Suppl 1):S12–9.

Urine Cytopathology and Ancillary Methods

Amy G. Zhou, MD, Lloyd M. Hutchinson, PhD, Ediz F. Cosar, MD*

KEYWORDS

- FISH • Urothelial carcinoma • Cytology • Molecular

ABSTRACT

Urothelial carcinoma (UC) is the most common malignancy of the urinary tract. Cytology and cystoscopy are two of the most commonly used tests for screening and diagnosis of UC. However, the sensitivity of cytology for UC is less than ideal, while cystoscopy is an invasive and expensive procedure. The search for an accurate, sensitive, noninvasive, and cost-effective method for detecting UC has led to the development of ancillary studies using immunological and molecular methods.

INTRODUCTION

Urothelial carcinoma (UC) is the most common malignancy of the urinary tract and accounts for more than 73,000 cases each year in the United States.[1] Cytology remains one of the most commonly used tests for the screening and diagnosis of UC, because it is both cost effective and noninvasive. Most often patients present with asymptomatic microhematuria, which is defined as 3 or more red blood cells per high-powered field on microscopy.[2] The most recent guideline from the American Urological Association (AUA) on the evaluation of asymptomatic microhematuria recommends a history, physical examination, urine culture, renal function tests, and imaging studies as an initial step. Cystoscopy is recommended for patients of age 35 or greater and in patients who have risk factors for genitourinary tract cancers. The AUA recommends that urine cytology and molecular tests be reserved for patients with persistent microhematuria whose initial work-up was negative or those who are at increased risk for UC.[2] In addition to its role in the initial diagnosis of UC, urine cytology has traditionally played an important part of monitoring for the recurrence of disease.

Urine cytology has a high sensitivity and specificity for the detection of high-grade UC but performs far from ideally when it comes to low-grade UC. A meta-analysis revealed that cytology has an overall sensitivity of 42% and specificity of 96% for UC,[3] including a sensitivity of approximately 30% for low-grade UC and 80% for high-grade UC.[4,5] Cystoscopy, however, is sensitive for low-grade papillary lesions but tends to miss urothelial carcinoma in situ (CIS), with an overall specificity of 88%.[6] Urine cytology and cystoscopy, therefore, seem to complement each other and have been widely used for initial diagnosis and follow-up of UC patients.[7] Cystoscopy is an invasive and expensive procedure, however, and the search for an accurate, sensitive, noninvasive, and cost-effective method for detecting UC continues to be at the frontier of scientific research.

Department of Pathology, University of Massachusetts Medical School, Three Biotech, One Innovation Drive, Worcester, MA 01605, USA
* Corresponding author.
E-mail address: Ediz.Cosar@umassmemorial.org

surgpath.theclinics.com

Key Points
UROTHELIAL CARCINOMA

The incidence of bladder cancer is more than 73,000 per year in the United States.

Bladder cancer causes more than 14,000 deaths per year in the United States.

More than 90% of bladder cancers in the United States are of urothelial origin.

A majority of UCs are low grade (80%).

Low-grade UC has a recurrence rate of 70%.

UC is more common in men, with a male:female ratio of 3:1.

UC is more common in patients greater than 50 years old.

Risk factors for UC include tobacco smoking, aniline dyes, phenacetin, and arsenic exposure.

UC usually presents with painless gross hematuria and may present with urgency or dysuria.

Cytologic Features of UC

Low Grade	High Grade
Increased nuclear-cytoplasmic (N/C) ratio	Markedly increased N/C ratio
Homogeneous cytoplasm	Nuclear hyperchromasia
Uniform granular chromatin	Coarse granular chromatin
Irregular nuclear contour	Irregular nuclear contour
Small distinct nucleoli	Large nucleoli
Umbrella cells variable	Umbrella cells absent
Mitoses infrequent	Mitoses frequent
Papillary fragments possible	More often single cells

CYTOLOGIC DIFFERENTIAL DIAGNOSIS

Urine cytology is the microscopic examination of exfoliated cells from the urinary tract into the urine, which may come from the renal pelvis, ureters, bladder, or urethra, all of which are normally lined by urothelium. The major purpose of urine cytology in clinical practice is to identify or rule out a neoplastic process, most commonly UC. UC is divided into low-grade and high-grade categories based on cytologic features. The diagnostic sensitivity of urine cytology and agreement among cytopathologists for high-grade UC is relatively high, whereas it is suboptimal for the detection of low-grade UC.[8]

Reactive changes are commonly seen in association with conditions that result in injury to the urothelium, such as acute or chronic cystitis, renal calculi, and instrumentation, which must be differentiated from neoplastic cells (**Table 1**).[8] Polyomavirus frequently produces enlarged cells (known as decoy cells) with ground-glass nuclei, intranuclear viral inclusions, and increased N/C ratio, which may be mistaken for high-grade UC. Upper urinary tract brushings or washings also often contain cells with large nuclei with prominent nucleoli, which occasionally may be mistaken for neoplastic cells.[8] Bilateral washings can sometimes help clarify the significance of these cells, because tumor is less likely to be bilateral.

Although uncommon, malignancies, such as renal cell carcinoma and prostatic adenocarcinoma, may shed tumor cells into urine. Other rare malignancies of the urinary tract include primary small cell carcinoma, squamous cell carcinoma, lymphomas, and sarcomas. Although these rare malignancies may have distinct cytologic features, occasionally they may pose a challenge to pathologists, because they can mimic a high-grade UC in appearance.

Pitfalls
OF CYTOLOGY

! Ureteral washings and brushings are more cellular and show higher N/C ratio, which may lead to a false-positive diagnosis. Bilateral washings may be helpful in these cases.

! Urine in bacillus Calmette-Guérin (BCG) patients may have cells with increased atypia and hyperchromasia, but N/C ratio is usually not increased. Other therapies, such as radiation or mitomycin C chemotherapy, may show similar effects.

! The nuclear changes in low-grade UC may be subtle and difficult to differentiate from normal urothelial cells.

! Instrumentation, stones, and viruses (cytomegalovirus and polyomavirus) may cause changes that mimic UC, especially high-grade UC.

Table 1
Cytologic differential diagnosis of urothelial carcinoma

	LG UC	HG UC	Reactive	Calculi	Polyomavirus	Post-Therapy	Instrumentation
Cellularity	High	High	Modest	Medium	Variable	Variable	High
Cytoplasm	Opaque	Variable	Abundant	Frayed	Scant	Variable	Textured
Nucleus size	Larger	Large	Increased	Variable	Large	Large	Normal
Nucleus shape	Oval, irregular	Irregular	Round, oval	Irregular	Round	Irregular	Round
Nucleoli	Absent	Variable	Prominent	Variable	Absent	Prominent	Tiny
Chromatin	Uniform, darker	Dark, irregular	Granular, uniform	Dark, coarse	Ground glass, marginated	Variable, dark	Pale, uniform
N/C ratio	Increased	High	Moderate	Variable	High	Moderate	Normal
Background	Clean	Variable	Inflamed	Dirty	Variable	Inflamed	Clean

Abbreviations: HG, high grade; LG, low grade.
Modified from Rosenthal D, Raab SS. Cytologic detection of urothelial lesions. New York: Springer; 2006; with permission.

There are several limitations of urine cytology as a diagnostic tool. First, low-grade UC is difficult to diagnose by cytology and is responsible for the low overall sensitivity of the test. Secondly, urine cytology does not help pinpoint the exact location of an urothelial lesion. In cases where no lesion is identified on cystoscopy but urine is positive for malignancy, radiologic imaging becomes of paramount importance in locating the lesion. Third, other cell types (ie, squamous cells or blood) or debris may contaminate a urine specimen (in particular voided urine specimens) and obscure the cells of importance. Lastly, there is a great deal of interobserver variability among cytopathologists in diagnosing UC,[9] especially low-grade type.

ANCILLARY STUDIES

Immunocytochemistry (ICC) is rarely used in the cytologic diagnosis of UC. In rare instances where a metastatic tumor enters the differential diagnosis, however, ICC may be helpful in determining the origin of the tumor, especially if biopsy material is not available.[10]

Many ancillary studies have been studied and developed over recent years in an attempt to improve the diagnostic accuracy of urine specimens. Food and Drug Administration (FDA)-approved urine-based methods include UroVysion (Abbott Laboratories, Abbott Park, Illinois) fluorescence in situ hybridization (FISH), bladder tumor antigen (BTA), nuclear matrix protein 22 (NMP22) (Alere Scarborough Inc., Scarborough, Maine), and immunocytology.

IMMUNOLOGY-BASED METHODS

There are several immunology-based methods of detecting UC (**Table 2**). This discussion is limited to those approved by the FDA, namely Immuno-Cyt, BTA, and NMP22.

Immunocyt is a fluorescent microscope-based test and is a method of detecting tumor-related antigens in urine specimens. It is a fluorescence immunoassay that uses antibodies against 3 antigens commonly expressed by UC cells (M344, LDQ10, and 19A211). M344 and LDQ10 are 2 mucin-like proteins, whereas 19A211 is a high-molecular-weight form of carcinoembryonic antigen. M344 and LDQ10 are expressed in 71% of stage pTa and pT1 UCs, whereas 19A211 is expressed in 90% of pTa and pT1 UCs.[11] The overall assay sensitivity and specificity are 81% and 75%, respectively,[12] and the assay is equally good at detecting both high-grade and low-grade UC. Disadvantages of Immunocyt include high cost and the need for 500 cells for a negative diagnosis, which is labor intensive, requiring extensive training for technicians and pathologists. False-positive results (21%)[13] are often caused by hematuria and other inflammatory processes, such as urinary tract infection, and BCG treatment.[14]

BTA TRAK (Polymedco Inc., Cortlandt Manor, NY) is a BTA assay that detects the human complement factor H (hCFH)-related protein (hCFHrp) in urine that is usually present in high concentrations in the urine of UC patients. BTA TRAK is an ELISA that is performed in the laboratory and can be a helpful adjunct to urine cytology. The sensitivity of this assay is approximately 69% and the

Table 2
Ancillary studies

Method	Sensitivity (%)	Specificity (%)	Comment
FDA approved			
Cytology	42	96	Low sensitivity for low-grade UC
FISH	72	83	Low but improved sensitivity for low-grade UC
Target-FISH	70	93	Improves specificity of FISH
Immunocyt	81	75	Technically simple but interpretation is challenging
BTA TRAK	69	65	Low specificity
BTA *stat*	70	75	Low specificity
NMP22 Bladderchek	50	87	Low sensitivity
Not FDA approved			
Lewis X antigen	83	85	—
BLCA-1	80	87	—
BLCA-4	89	100	—
Survivin	64–94	93–100	—
Microsatellite analysis	85	90	—
Telomerase	70–90	80–90	—
Quanticyt nuclear karyometry	60	70	—
Hyaluronic acid	91	84	—
Aurora kinase A	87	97	—

Data from Refs.[3,12,14,44]

specificity is 65%, and it is much better at detecting high-grade UC (sensitivity 75%) than low-grade UC (sensitivity 45%–60%).[15] Conditions causing hematuria, such as urinary tract infection or bladder stones, may lead to false-positive results in approximately 25% of cases,[15] because hCFH from blood is detected instead.[12] The BTA *stat* (Polymedco Inc., Cortlandt Manor, NY) Test is a qualitative point-of-care counterpart assay, often used in urologists' offices, which is reportedly more accurate and has 70% sensitivity and 75% specificity.[12]

The NMP22 Test is an assay for the NMP22, which plays a regulatory role in mitosis during cell division. There is an ELISA form of this assay that is associated with a high false-positive rate of 36%[15] and, therefore, not often used. The BladderChek is a dipstick test, used as a point-of-care test in physician offices, which has median sensitivity and specificity of 50% and 87%, respectively.[12] False-positive results (24%)[15] are often related to inflammation, stones, and hematuria.[12]

Key Points
IMMUNOLOGY-BASED ASSAYS

Immunocytology

Detects tumor-associated antigens M344, LDQ10, and 19A211

Requires fluorescent microscope to examine cells

BTA *stat* and BTA TRAK

Detect complement factor H–related protein in voided urine

ELISA or point-of-care tests

NMP22 Test

Detects a nuclear mitotic apparatus protein in voided urine

Seems unaffected by BCG therapy

ELISA or point-of-care test

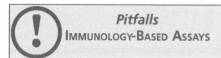

MOLECULAR TESTING

One of the first genetic alterations usually occurs in chromosome 9, involving p16, located at the 9p21 locus, as well as mutations in other potential tumor suppressor genes on chromosome 9, such as TSC1, DBC1, PTCH1, MSSE, and CDKN1B.[16] Mutations in chromosome 9 are followed by divergent pathways of additional genetic defects (**Fig. 1**).[17] It is now known that low-grade papillary UC tends to involve activating mutations in the HRAS, FGFR3,

and PIK3CA genes, which promote cell growth in UC. High-grade and muscle-invasive UC tends to harbor alterations in the p53 and Rb tumor suppressor genes involved in cell cycle control.[18] MDM2 amplification is also found in high-grade UC, whereas loss of PTEN is commonly associated with muscle-invasive disease.[19]

Armed with the knowledge from molecular studies, a variety of methods have been developed over recent years in an attempt to improve the diagnostic accuracy of UC in urine specimens. The only FDA-approved urine-based molecular method is UroVysion FISH, which incorporates a probe to detect 9p21 defects. Commercial FISH probes are also available for other genes (eg, TP53, PTEN, and MDM2). FISH analysis of these genes or testing for recurrent mutations (eg, FGFR3) is, however, not yet part of routine clinical practice.

FISH

UroVysion is FDA approved in voided urine for both new diagnosis of UC and for follow-up of patients with a history of UC. Other specimen types require laboratory validation. This multitarget, multicolor FISH assay (4-probe set) examines the more common chromosomal abnormalities in UC using centromeric fluorescent denatured chromosome enumeration probes for chromosomes 3, 7, and 17 and a locus-specific identifier probe for 9p21. Normal cells are disomic with this probe set, whereas genetic abnormalities observed in

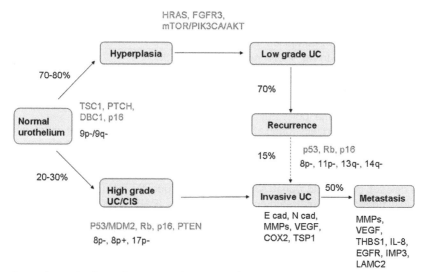

Fig. 1. Molecular pathways in the pathogenesis of UC. (*Modified from* Wu XR. Urothelial tumorigenesis: a tale of divergent pathways. Nat Rev Cancer 2005;5:716; with permission.)

UC include polysomy (including tetrasomy), trisomy, and 9p21 deletion.

In a meta-analysis study, the sensitivity and specificity of FISH were 72% and 83%, respectively.[3] Similar to cytology, FISH is more sensitive in detecting high-grade UC (including CIS) compared with low-grade UC.[20] The sensitivity of FISH for high-grade UC is 81% to 100%[20,21] compared with 48% for low-grade UC.[20] The FDA-approved criteria for a positive FISH result include (1) 4 or more cells with polysomy (3 or more copies of 2 or more chromosomes) or (2) 9p21 homozygous deletion in 12 or more cells. Although a minimum of 25 morphologically abnormal cells needs to be scanned, many laboratories use automation to scan hundreds of cells to decrease the likelihood of overlooking a tumor cell.

FISH is most useful in cases of equivocal cytology, which can help clinicians identify those patients who may need further work-up, such as cystoscopy and biopsy. Urine specimens classified as atypical or suspicious for malignancy may benefit from prompt reflex FISH testing to provide a more definitive diagnosis[22] of UC. This strategy has also been shown cost effective.[23] Advantages of FISH include that it is a noninvasive procedure, it has higher sensitivity compared with cytology,[24] and its accuracy is not affected by hematuria or other inflammatory processes, such as urinary tract infection and BCG treatment.[25] FISH is also able to detect rare types of bladder cancer, such as squamous cell carcinoma (approximately 20%) and adenocarcinoma (approximately 80%).[26]

FISH has several disadvantages. This method is an expensive and time-consuming test and requires a fluorescent microscope, specially trained technicians to perform the assay, and molecular pathologists to render interpretations. Pitfalls associated with interpretation of FISH results include the detection of chromosome tetrasomy (a natural product of cell division) and reduced specificity of FISH to predict recurrence of disease if tetrasomy is included in the polysomy category.[27] In addition, technical artifacts often associated with poor preservation of cells may adversely affect interpretation of FISH signals. For instance, poor hybridization of the 9p21 probe may be misinterpreted as deletion of the gold signal. Atypical cells may be lost during FISH pretreatment and hybridization steps reducing the likelihood of detecting tumor cells. Although not included in the original FDA-approved criteria, gain of a single chromosome or hemizygous loss of 9p21[28,29] may be the only abnormality detected in low-grade UC.

Key Points
FISH

FISH is FDA approved for follow-up of patients with a history of UC and for new diagnosis of UC in patients with hematuria.

FDA criteria for positive FISH are 4 or more cells with polysomy (3 or more copies of 2 or more chromosomes) or 9p21 homozygous deletion in 12 or more cells.

A minimum of 25 morphologically abnormal cells needs to be scanned.

Pitfalls
OF FISH

! Tetrasomy cells are the product of natural cell division and, when included in the polysomy category, lead to false-positive results.

! Polyploidization is frequently seen in umbrella cells and may mimic a positive FISH result.

! Technical artifacts resulting in poor signal quality may be misinterpreted as homozygous loss of 9p21.

! Dark-field microscopy may fail to evaluate rare atypical urothelial cells, potentially leading to a false-negative result.

! FISH-only approach without integrating cytology has limited value in identifying the cell or tumor type.

! Cells of interest may be lost during processing.

PRACTICAL APPLICATIONS

Ideally, a combination of cytology and FISH is used for the detection of bladder cancer, using bright-field microscopy to select atypical cells that are then targeted for FISH. Pathologists are subsequently able to compare bright-field Papanicolaou (PAP) stain and fluorescent views of the same cell and simultaneously use morphology and FISH to improve the diagnostic accuracy. This methodology helps decrease the number of false-positive results by excluding nonurothelial cells or benign umbrella cells that may show an abnormal FISH signal. Using this combined approach (target-FISH), FISH has a sensitivity of approximately 66% (87.5% for high-grade UC and 44.6% for low-grade UC) and specificity of 93.7%. Examples are shown in **Figs. 2–4**.

Although a helpful test for the diagnosis of UC, FISH does not necessarily have to be done for all patients for whom UC is suspected. Patients with positive cytology do not need to have FISH performed given the high specificity of cytology for UC. Reflex testing of target-FISH is recommended for clarifying suspicious or atypical urine cytology diagnoses. A study showed that 91% of patients with positive FISH and equivocal cytology were found to have UC on subsequent biopsy.[30] The sensitivity of FISH for UC in suspicious, atypical, and negative cytology cases is 100%, 89%,

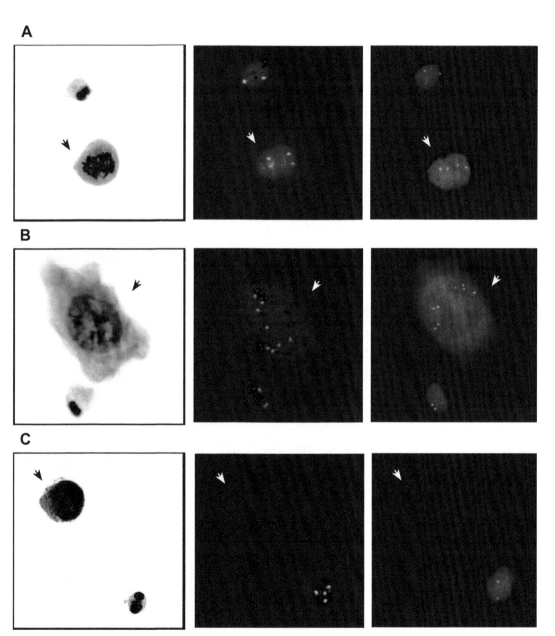

Fig. 2. Pitfalls of standard FISH may be clarified using Target-FISH. PAP-stained urine cytology and FISH abnormalities for chromosomes 3 (*red*), 7 (*green*), 17 (*aqua*), and 9p21 (*gold*). (*A*) Dividing urothelial cell with 4 signals for each probe (*arrow*), with a neutrophil nearby showing disomy for all 4 chromosome probes. Tetrasomy is a natural product of cell division and should be excluded from polysomy category. (*B*) Umbrella cell showing octosomy (*arrow*). (*C*) Loss of atypical cell during processing of FISH slides, indicated by arrow.

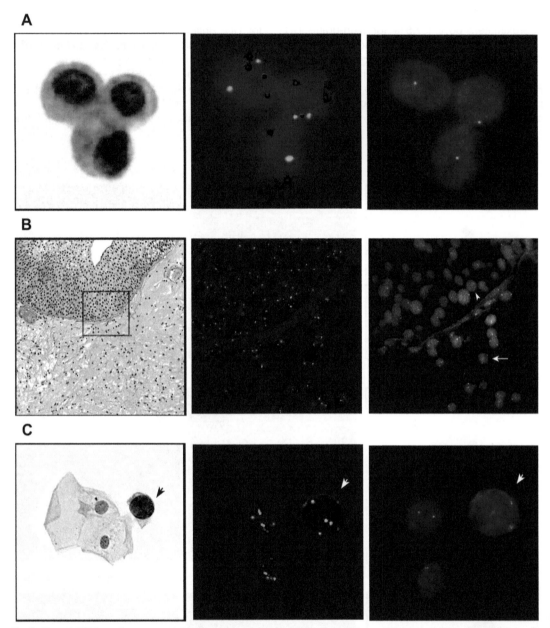

Fig. 3. Target FISH can improve sensitivity and specificity. PAP-stained urine cytology and FISH abnormalities for chromosomes 3 (*red*), 7 (*green*), 17 (*aqua*), and 9p21 (*gold*). (*A*) Atypical cytology, low-grade UC with hemizygous loss of 9p21 (1 gold signal). (*B*) This was confirmed on the surgical specimen, depicted as hematoxylin-eosin (10) with magnified area (*box*) showing normal diploid cells (*arrow*) and tumor cells with hemizygous loss of 9p21 (*arrowhead*). (*C*) Atypical cells seen in polyomavirus infection are mostly disomic and show two copies of each FISH signal (*arrow*).

and 60% respectively.[31] In the authors' experience, a suspicious cytology diagnosis is associated with a positive biopsy in 60% of patients, suggesting that FISH may be helpful in selecting patients for cystoscopy. Another study showed that the sensitivity of FISH is much higher (65%)

in patients with a greater than 40 pack-year smoking history compared with nonsmokers (13.6%) and those with a 20- to 40-year smoking history (24.2%).[20] This suggests that FISH may be more appropriate for patients with a high pretest probability of having UC, such as patients age 45 or

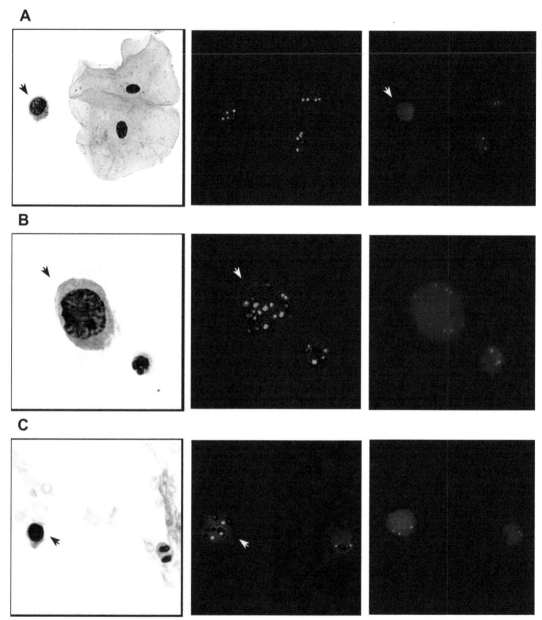

Fig. 4. Common abnormalities seen in bladder tumors. PAP-stained urine cytology and FISH abnormalities for chromosomes 3 (*red*), 7 (*green*), 17 (*aqua*), and 9p21 (*gold*). (*A*) Atypical urine cytology, low-grade UC with homozygous loss of 9p21 (*gold*), indicated by arrow. (*B*) Urine cytology, suspicious for malignancy (*arrow*); high-grade UC with chromosome polysomy (*arrow*). (*C*) Small cell carcinoma with chromosome polysomy (*arrow*). Target-FISH aids in cell classification.

older[25] with a smoking history. A proposed algorithm for the use of FISH is shown in **Fig. 5**.

FISH is useful in follow-up of UC patients, because it has been shown to detect recurrence of UC several months in advance of a positive cystoscopy or biopsy. This is sometimes known as "anticipatory positive" finding. In a surveillance study of UC patients, 65% of patients who had a positive FISH but negative cytology and biopsy developed recurrent disease within 29 months.[32] This makes FISH a useful surveillance tool for the detection of recurrent UC.

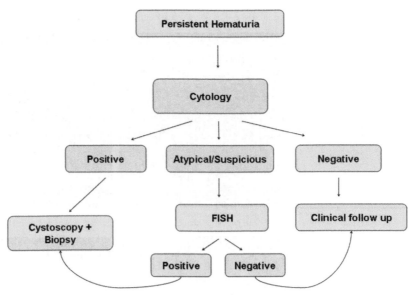

Fig. 5. Proposed diagnostic algorithm for persistent hematuria.

Practical Applications FISH

FISH is approved for use with voided urine. Other specimen types (such as upper tract washings) can be used but require validation.

FISH is not indicated for all hematuria patients. It has a higher positive predictive value for patients greater than age 45 with a smoking history.

FISH is useful as an adjunct to cystoscopy and cytology, especially in the case of equivocal cytology results.

FISH results may be "anticipatory positive" months before a positive cystoscopy or biopsy result.

FISH is typically not affected by polyomavirus or BCG treatment and is a reliable indicator of recurrence.

THERAPEUTIC AND PROGNOSTIC APPLICATIONS

Tumor stage is the major prognostic factor in UC. Other risk factors include grade, tumor size, multifocality, presence of CIS,[7] and increased Ki-67 proliferation index.[17] The genetics of tumorigenesis in UC is complex, and studies have demonstrated associations between various genetic markers and prognosis. Patients with a positive FISH after BCG therapy have a 2.7 to 4.6 times higher risk of tumor recurrence compared with FISH-negative patients and may also have an increased risk of muscle invasive disease.[33–35] Using FISH, it has been suggested that the percentage of abnormal cells predicts cancer recurrence and progression to invasive disease.[33] The results from these studies are mainly in research stages and not used routinely for clinical prognostication of patients.

FUTURE TRENDS

Recent studies on fibroblast growth factor receptor (FGFR) show promising results. Activating mutations of FGFR3 are present in approximately half of all UCs and approximately 70% of noninvasive low-grade papillary UCs.[36] FGFR3 is a receptor tyrosine kinase that plays a role in intracellular signaling, and mutations are likely responsible for increased growth signals that lead to tumorigenesis. These tumors are less likely to progress to muscle invasive disease, yielding a more favorable prognosis.[37] FGFR3 mutation analysis may be useful as a urine biomarker for diagnosis and detecting recurrence in UC patients.[37] Hotspot mutations identified in FGFR3 can be detected by PCR techniques with high sensitivity. Because the FGFR3 mutation is often present in low-grade UC, it may be a valuable adjunct to cytology, particularly in situations where baseline FISH is negative. A recent study showed adding FGFR3 analysis to cytology improved sensitivity from

53% to 73%.[38] Further studies are necessary before these methods are introduced into standard clinical practice.

Other emerging topics of interest include micro-RNAs that are regularly up-regulated or down-regulated in UC,[39] which may become a useful diagnostic tool. Researchers screened for mutations in genes commonly involved in UC tumorigenesis (ie, FGFR3, TP53, and HRAS) and combined this with methylation status to form a panel of markers for the detection of UC.[40] Recent studies have identified mutations in the promoter region of the telomerase reverse transcriptase (TERT) gene in urothelial tumors with high frequency.[41] TERT mutations occur early in the tumorigenesis of 66% of muscle invasive UC and 74% of noninvasive UC.[42] These findings are promising for a urine-based TERT mutation assay for the detection and follow up of UC in the near future. Massively parallel sequencing (next-generation sequencing) has potential to act as a universal platform to look at multiple molecular abnormalities simultaneously. In the near future, this may lead to comprehensive profiling of each tumor even without the need for a biopsy and allow for individualized targeted therapies.[43]

REFERENCES

1. Siegel R, Naishadham D, Jemal A. Cancer statistics, 2012. CA Cancer J Clin 2012;62:10–29.
2. Davis R, Jones JS, Barocas DA, et al. Diagnosis, evaluation and follow-up of asymptomatic microhematuria (AMH) in adults: AUA guideline. J Urol 2012;188:2473–81.
3. Hajdinjak T. UroVysion FISH test for detecting urothelial cancers: meta-analysis of diagnostic accuracy and comparison with urinary cytology testing. Urol Oncol 2008;26:646–51.
4. Bastacky S, Ibrahim S, Wilczynski SP, et al. The accuracy of urinary cytology in daily practice. Cancer 1999;87:118–28.
5. Renshaw AA, Nappi D, Weinberg DS. Cytology of grade 1 papillary transitional cell carcinoma. A comparison of cytologic, architectural and morphometric criteria in cystoscopically obtained urine. Acta Cytol 1996;40:676–82.
6. Schlake A, Crispen PL, Cap AP, et al. NMP-22, urinary cytology, and cystoscopy: a 1 year comparison study. Can J Urol 2012;19:6345–50.
7. Prasad SM, Decastro GJ, Steinberg GD. Urothelial carcinoma of the bladder: definition, treatment and future efforts. Nat Rev Urol 2011;8:631–42.
8. Flezar MS. Urine and bladder washing cytology for detection of urothelial carcinoma: standard test with new possibilities. Radiol Oncol 2010;44:207–14.
9. Owens CL, Vandenbussche CJ, Burroughs FH, et al. A review of reporting systems and terminology for urine cytology. Cancer Cytopathol 2013;121:9–14.
10. Srivastava R, Arora VK, Aggarwal S, et al. Cytokeratin-20 immunocytochemistry in voided urine cytology and its comparison with nuclear matrix protein-22 and urine cytology in the detection of urothelial carcinoma. Diagn Cytopathol 2012;40:755–9.
11. Vrooman OP, Witjes JA. Urinary markers in bladder cancer. Eur Urol 2008;53:909–16.
12. Wadhwa N, Jatawa SK, Tiwari A. Non-invasive urine based tests for the detection of bladder cancer. J Clin Pathol 2012;65:970–5.
13. Mian C, Pycha A, Wiener H, et al. Immunocyt: a new tool for detecting transitional cell cancer of the urinary tract. J Urol 1999;161:1486–9.
14. Tetu B. Diagnosis of urothelial carcinoma from urine. Mod Pathol 2009;22(Suppl 2):S53–9.
15. van Rhijn BW, van der Poel HG, van der Kwast TH. Urine markers for bladder cancer surveillance: a systematic review. Eur Urol 2005;47:736–48.
16. Al Hussain TO, Akhtar M. Molecular basis of urinary bladder cancer. Adv Anat Pathol 2013;20:53–60.
17. Netto GJ. Molecular diagnostics in urologic malignancies: a work in progress. Arch Pathol Lab Med 2011;135:610–21.
18. Netto GJ, Cheng L. Emerging critical role of molecular testing in diagnostic genitourinary pathology. Arch Pathol Lab Med 2012;136:372–90.
19. McConkey DJ, Lee S, Choi W, et al. Molecular genetics of bladder cancer: emerging mechanisms of tumor initiation and progression. Urol Oncol 2010;28:429–40.
20. Sarosdy MF, Kahn PR, Ziffer MD, et al. Use of a multitarget fluorescence in situ hybridization assay to diagnose bladder cancer in patients with hematuria. J Urol 2006;176:44–7.
21. Halling KC, King W, Sokolova IA, et al. A comparison of cytology and fluorescence in situ hybridization for the detection of urothelial carcinoma. J Urol 2000;164:1768–75.
22. Lotan Y, Bensalah K, Ruddell T, et al. Prospective evaluation of the clinical usefulness of reflex fluorescence in situ hybridization assay in patients with atypical cytology for the detection of urothelial carcinoma of the bladder. J Urol 2008;179:2164–9.
23. Gayed BA, Seideman C, Lotan Y. Cost-effectiveness of fluorescence in situ hybridization in patients with atypical cytology for the detection of urothelial carcinoma. J Urol 2013;190(4):1181–6.
24. Arentsen HC, de la Rosette JJ, de Reijke TM, et al. Fluorescence in situ hybridization: a multitarget approach in diagnosis and management of urothelial cancer. Expert Rev Mol Diagn 2007;7:11–9.

25. Halling KC, Kipp BR. Bladder cancer detection using FISH (UroVysion assay). Adv Anat Pathol 2008;15:279–86.

26. Reid-Nicholson MD, Ramalingam P, Adeagbo B, et al. The use of Urovysion fluorescence in situ hybridization in the diagnosis and surveillance of non-urothelial carcinoma of the bladder. Mod Pathol 2009;22:119–27.

27. Zellweger T, Benz G, Cathomas G, et al. Multi-target fluorescence in situ hybridization in bladder washings for prediction of recurrent bladder cancer. Int J Cancer 2006;119:1660–5.

28. Bubendorf L, Grilli B, Sauter G, et al. Multiprobe FISH for enhanced detection of bladder cancer in voided urine specimens and bladder washings. Am J Clin Pathol 2001;116:79–86.

29. Zhou AG, Garver J, Woda BA, et al. The Utility of Relative Loss of 9p21 In UroVysion Fluorescence In Situ Hybridization (FISH) for The Detection Of Urothelial Carcinoma (UC) [CAP Abstract 106]. Arch Pathol Lab Med 2013;137:1512.

30. Kipp BR, Halling KC, Campion MB, et al. Assessing the value of reflex fluorescence in situ hybridization testing in the diagnosis of bladder cancer when routine urine cytological examination is equivocal. J Urol 2008;179:1296–301 [discussion: 301].

31. Skacel M, Fahmy M, Brainard JA, et al. Multitarget fluorescence in situ hybridization assay detects transitional cell carcinoma in the majority of patients with bladder cancer and atypical or negative urine cytology. J Urol 2003;169:2101–5.

32. Yoder BJ, Skacel M, Hedgepeth R, et al. Reflex UroVysion testing of bladder cancer surveillance patients with equivocal or negative urine cytology: a prospective study with focus on the natural history of anticipatory positive findings. Am J Clin Pathol 2007;127:295–301.

33. Kipp BR, Tanasescu M, Else TA, et al. Quantitative fluorescence in situ hybridization and its ability to predict bladder cancer recurrence and progression to muscle-invasive bladder cancer. J Mol Diagn 2009;11:148–54.

34. Kipp BR, Karnes RJ, Brankley SM, et al. Monitoring intravesical therapy for superficial bladder cancer using fluorescence in situ hybridization. J Urol 2005;173:401–4.

35. Mengual L, Marin-Aguilera M, Ribal MJ, et al. Clinical utility of fluorescent in situ hybridization for the surveillance of bladder cancer patients treated with bacillus Calmette-Guerin therapy. Eur Urol 2007;52:752–9.

36. Zuiverloon TC, van der Aa MN, van der Kwast TH, et al. Fibroblast growth factor receptor 3 mutation analysis on voided urine for surveillance of patients with low-grade non-muscle-invasive bladder cancer. Clin Cancer Res 2010;16:3011–8.

37. Zuiverloon TC, Tjin SS, Busstra M, et al. Optimization of nonmuscle invasive bladder cancer recurrence detection using a urine based FGFR3 mutation assay. J Urol 2011;186:707–12.

38. van Kessel KE, Kompier LC, de Bekker-Grob EW, et al. FGFR3 mutation analysis in voided urine samples to decrease cystoscopies and cost in nonmuscle invasive bladder cancer surveillance: a comparison of 3 strategies. J Urol 2013;189:1676–81.

39. Mengual L, Lozano JJ, Ingelmo-Torres M, et al. Using microRNA profiling in urine samples to develop a non-invasive test for bladder cancer. Int J Cancer 2013;133(11):2631–41.

40. Serizawa RR, Ralfkiaer U, Steven K, et al. Integrated genetic and epigenetic analysis of bladder cancer reveals an additive diagnostic value of FGFR3 mutations and hypermethylation events. Int J Cancer 2011;129:78–87.

41. Hurst CD, Platt FM, Knowles MA. Comprehensive Mutation Analysis of the TERT Promoter in Bladder Cancer and Detection of Mutations in Voided Urine. Eur Urol 2013. In press.

42. Papadopoulos N, Kinde I, Munari E, et al. TERT Promoter Mutations Occur Early in Urothelial Neoplasia and are Biomarkers of Early Disease and Disease Recurrence in Urine. Cancer Res 2013. In press.

43. Ross JS, Wang K, Al-Rohil RN, et al. Advanced urothelial carcinoma: next-generation sequencing reveals diverse genomic alterations and targets of therapy. Mod Pathol 2013. [Epub ahead of print].

44. Mitra AP, Cote RJ. Molecular pathogenesis and diagnostics of bladder cancer. Annu Rev Pathol 2009;4:251–85.

Ancillary Diagnostics in Gynecologic Cytology

Susanne Jeffus, MD[a], Kristen Atkins, MD[b],*

KEYWORDS

- Human papillomavirus • Hybrid capture • In situ hybridization • Squamous dysplasia
- Genomic testing

KEY POINTS

- The three main ways of detecting human papillomavirus are enhanced morphology though immunochemistry, detecting high risk HPV through hybrid capture, and identification of specific HPV types through genotyping.
- Immunochemistry for Ki67 and p16 assists in identifying high risk HPV through enhancing the morphologic evaluation of the Pap test.
- Management decisions are changing based on the genotyping identification of HPV 16 or 18.

ABSTRACT

Cytology has been the mainstay of cervical dysplasia and cancer screening in the United States. The specificity of a woman harboring a high-grade lesion when identified as high-grade squamous intraepithelial lesion on Pap test is high; however, the test suffers from low sensitivity. Epidemiology studies have demonstrated that human papillomavirus (HPV) types 16 and 18 account for most cervical squamous cell carcinomas. Tests have been developed to identify high-risk HPV, some specifically to identify HPV 16 and 18. Simultaneous to the increase in HPV detection methods, interdisciplinary groups are making recommendations on the managerial use of the tests.

INTRODUCTION

Cytology has been the mainstay of cervical dysplasia and cancer screening in the United States. Specimen collection is relatively easy and painless and the specificity of a woman harboring a high-grade lesion when identified as high-grade squamous intraepithelial lesion (HSIL) on Papanicolaou (Pap) test is very high. However, the Pap test suffers from a low sensitivity (50%–70%), and as such there has been an enormous effort to improve cervical screening tests and identify more women with high-grade lesions.[1] At the same time, large epidemiology studies have demonstrated that human papillomavirus (HPV) types 16 and 18 account for the vast majority of cervical squamous cell carcinomas, have the highest binding affinity to E6 and E7, are the most common persistent HPV infections, and tend to have the most rapid progression from infection to high-grade dysplasia to carcinoma.[2] As a result of the understanding of the biology of HPV infections, tests have been developed to identify high-risk HPV (hr-HPV) and some specifically to identify HPV 16 and HPV 18. These tests have come in the form of (1) morphologic enhancement via immunohistochemistry and in situ hybridization, (2) detection of pooled hr-HPV through hybrid capture techniques, and (3) identification of specific HPV types through genotyping. Simultaneous to the increase in HPV detection methods, interdisciplinary groups are making recommendations on the managerial use of the tests and subsequent management (Table 1).[3]

[a] Department of Pathology, University of Arkansas Medical Sciences, 4301 W. Markham Street, Slot #517, Little Rock, AR 72205, USA; [b] Department of Pathology, University of Virginia, 1215 Lee Street, Office 3034, Charlottesville, VA 22908, USA
* Corresponding author.
E-mail address: Kaa2p@virginia.edu

Surgical Pathology 7 (2014) 89–103
http://dx.doi.org/10.1016/j.path.2013.10.002
1875-9181/14/$ – see front matter © 2014 Elsevier Inc. All rights reserved.

surgpath.theclinics.com

Table 1
Comparison of human papillomavirus (HPV) tests

	Immunocytochemistry	Hybrid Capture	Genotyping
Morphologic test	Yes	No	No
Specifically Identifies HPV 16 and 18	No	No	Yes
May cross-react with low-risk HPV	Yes	Yes	No

CYTOLOGIC DIFFERENTIAL DIAGNOSIS

In the United States, cervical morphology via the Pap test is still the most common initial screening test for the detection of cervical cancer and findings are uniformly reported by laboratories using the Bethesda System Terminology.[4] The most common abnormal cytologic diagnosis in the Pap test is "Atypical Squamous Cells" (ASC). About half of these diagnoses are secondary to reactive changes, but our ability to appropriately categorize them into reactive or HPV-related groups on morphology alone is poor.[5] The category "Atypical Squamous Cells, cannot exclude a high-grade lesion" (ASC-H) more often is associated with high-grade squamous intraepithelial lesion than ASC, but still most cases have tissue biopsies less than cervical intraepithelial neoplasia (CIN) 2.[6] Immature squamous metaplasia and atrophy are great mimickers of high-grade squamous intraepithelial lesion and are a common benign explanation of an ASC-H interpretation.[4]

All of the cytologic uncertainty is compounded by the great variability in the histologic diagnosis of CIN 2 on biopsy.[7] Additionally, the natural biology of CIN 2 is variable and not predictable on morphology alone. Some CIN 2 lesions will regress, some will persist, and some will progress to invasive carcinoma. The differential diagnosis of CIN 2 is often CIN 1 or CIN 3.

ANCILLARY STUDIES

IMMUNOCYTOCHEMISTRY AND IN-SITU HYBRIDIZATION

Immunocytochemical markers have been studied as an approach to identifying the presence of hr-HPV testing by using unstained slides or cell blocks from residual material from liquid-based Pap tests.[8,9] The benefits of immunocytochemistry are ease of implementation, low cost, and potential for automation. The most robust biomarkers evaluated in the cytology literature of HPV-induced intraepithelial lesions include $p16^{INK4a}$, Ki-67 (MIB-1), minichromosome maintenance protein 2 (MCM2), and DNA topoisomerase IIα (TOP2A), all used as stand-alone immunocytochemical markers or in combination. For a more extensive summary of immunocytochemical markers, the reader is referred to the review by Pinto and colleagues.[9]

$P16^{INK4A}$

$p16^{INK4a}$ (p16) is a surrogate marker for infection with hr-HPV. It is a prototypic INK4 protein whose function is to inhibit cyclin-dependent kinase-mediated phosphorylation of the retinoblastoma (Rb) gene product leading to downregulation of cell proliferation. In the setting of persistent infection with hr-HPV, the E7 oncoprotein binds to the host Rb protein, which results in the inactivation of Rb and release and subsequent activation of the transcription factor E2F. These actions commit the cell to division. Simultaneously, E2F causes a marked increase in the production of p16; however, its inhibitory effect on cell proliferation is lost. This paradoxic overexpression makes p16 a sensitive biomarker for HPV infections caused by hr-HPV types.[9]

The overexpression of p16 in the setting of HPV infection is evident by accumulation of the protein in the nucleus and cytoplasm. In histologic sections, strong and diffuse nuclear or nuclear plus cytoplasmic staining with p16 from the basal cell layer upward correlates well with the presence of an HSIL (**Fig. 1**).[10] In cervicovaginal samples, a positive immunocytochemical stain is demonstrated by brown cytoplasmic staining with slightly darker brown nuclear staining. p16 staining identifies cells that may be missed by standard screening alone. However, because p16 positivity also can be seen in tubal metaplasia, squamous metaplasia, endometrial cells, and Trichomonas, interpretation of the stain requires correlation with the appropriate cytomorphologic criteria of dysplasia.[11–14]

Fig. 1. Hematoxylin and eosin (H&E) section of a cervical biopsy in which high-grade squamous intraepithelial lesion (CIN2) was questioned (*A*, original magnification ×400). A p16 immunohistochemical stain demonstrated strong confluent positivity supporting an HSIL diagnosis (*B*, original magnification ×100).

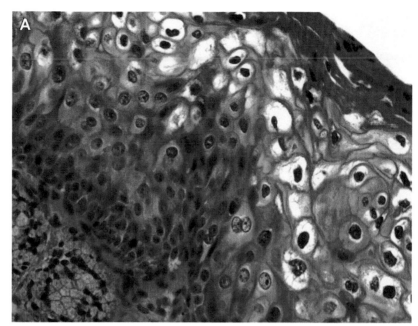

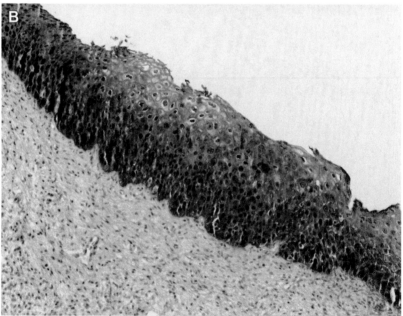

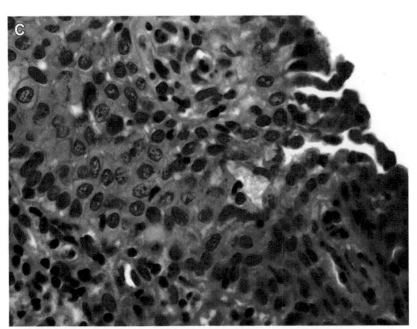

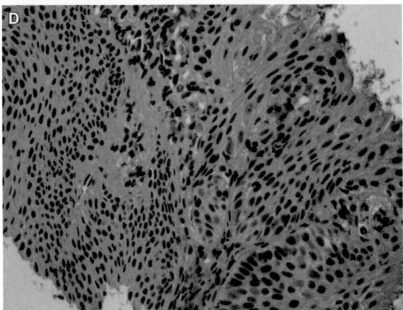

Fig. 1. H&E of a cervical biopsy with the differential diagnosis of squamous metaplasia versus HSIL (*C*, original magnification ×400). A p16 stain is negative supporting metaplasia (*D*, original magnification ×200).

THERAPEUTIC AND PROGNOSTIC APPLICATIONS OF P16^{INK4A}

Among the candidate immunomarkers for the detection of precancerous HPV-related lesions, p16 is the most studied biomarker. In tissue sections, p16 has been shown to improve interobserver agreement.[13,15,16] According to the Lower Anogenital Squamous Terminology Standardization Project (LAST) recommendations of Working group 4, only p16 had sufficient literature evidence to warrant its use as an adjunct biomarker for the diagnosis of HSIL.[17] Data regarding other biomarkers, including ProExC and Ki-67 (Mib-1), were insufficient for a recommendation regarding their utility for use alone or in combination with other biomarkers.[17]

Most collected data on the performance of p16 shows that when applied to liquid-based cytology or cell block preparations, p16 immunostaining improves the detection of HSIL over cytology alone.[9] In a meta-analysis of 61 studies by Tsoumpou and colleagues,[18] the investigators concluded that p16 overexpression correlated well with the severity of preneoplastic lesions in cytology and tissue sections. Denton and colleagues[19] evaluated p16 staining in cytology specimens in the largest retrospective study to date involving 810 cases of Atypical squamous cells of uncertain significance (ASC-US) and LSIL cytology. Their findings confirmed the data of smaller studies in that p16 showed similar sensitivity but improved specificity compared with molecular HPV (HC2) testing. In the most recent review and meta-analysis by Roelens and colleagues[20] of 17 major international studies, p16 immunocytochemistry, when compared with molecular testing (HC2), provided better specificity and comparable sensitivity in a cohort of 1740 women with ASC-US. With respect to triage of 2019 women with LSIL, p16 was less sensitive but more specific than molecular HPV testing.[20] Hence, p16 may represent an alternative triage approach of cytology specimens with mild abnormalities.

PRACTICAL APPLICATIONS OF P16[INK4A]

The role of p16 in cervical cancer screening requires larger prospective studies and a standardized immunocytochemical processing. Staining of bacteria and obscuring inflammatory cells as well as strong background staining can also prohibit the interpretative ease of p16.[14] These pitfalls, as well as the lack of a standardized scoring system for the interpretation of p16, have so far limited its routine application in the practice of cytology. p16 as a stand-alone immunocytochemical stain is not as practical as the combined p16/Ki-67 staining described later in this article (CINtec+).

KI-67 (MIB-1)

Ki-67 is a marker of cell proliferation and is expressed in all phases of the cell cycle. MIB-1 is a monoclonal antibody directed against the antigen Ki-67. It is a nuclear stain. As HPV infection results in an increase in the cell proliferation index, MIB-1 has been studied as a potential biomarker. In comparison with p16 and ProEx C, MIB-1 demonstrates a lower sensitivity and specificity for the detection of HSIL.[21–24] However, its value is most promising in combination with p16 (CINtec+ dual stain) as discussed in the next section.

CINTEC+: DUAL P16/KI-67 STAINING

Dual staining of cytology specimens with the surrogate marker for hr-HPV infection, p16, and the proliferation marker Ki-67 identifies replicating cells that have the potential for malignant transformation. Regardless of morphology, the dual staining highlights cells in which HPV has most likely integrated into the host genome leading to genetic instability and deregulation of the cell cycle.[25] Positive dual staining is virtually never found in normal suprabasal squamous cells, endocervical cells, or endometrial cells. This results in a high specificity and limits pitfalls encountered with p16 staining or Ki 67 staining alone.[26,27]

Currently, CINtec+ (Roche Labs formerly owned by mtm laboratories, Roche Diagnostics Corporation Indianapolis, Indiana) markets the dual stain p16/Ki-67. In liquid-based cytology specimens, a positive dual stain is defined as the presence of at least 1 cell demonstrating simultaneous brown cytoplasmic p16 and red nuclear Ki-67 staining (Fig. 2). Of note, this dual-staining pattern is to be interpreted as positive regardless of the presence or absence of morphologic alterations. The advantage of the dual stain is threefold: (1) identification of cells that may be missed through standard cervical screening improving the overall sensitivity of the Pap test, (2) ease of interpretation due to disregard of the morphologic criteria decreasing interobserver variability, and (3) circumvention of interpretative pitfalls (staining of normal glandular cells, tubal metaplasia) encountered with sole p16 staining.

THERAPEUTIC AND PROGNOSTIC APPLICATIONS OF CINTEC+ (DUAL P16/KI-67 STAINING)

Studies evaluating the utility of CINtec+ in the triage of cervical cancer screening are limited but promising. A recently published retrospective study by Schmidt and colleagues[25] evaluated the utility of dual staining for liquid-based cytology for the categories of ASC-US and LSIL using the same patient cohort as the p16 study by Denton and colleagues.[19] Schmidt and colleagues[25] found that dual staining identified HSIL with high sensitivity and even better specificity than with sole p16 immunocytochemical staining. Particularly in the ASC-US cohort, dual staining performed similarly to hr-HPV testing for the triage of women to colposcopy. Further data support that dual staining carries a high sensitivity and improved specificity over hr-HPV testing or sole p16 immunocytochemical staining and may represent a novel cervical cancer screening approach.[28–33]

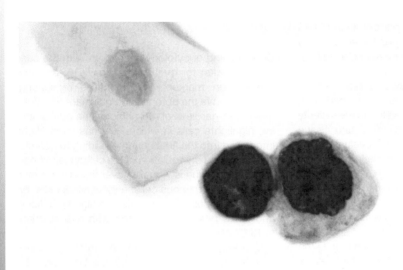

Fig. 2. Dual p16 and Ki67 staining showing the positive cytoplasmic and nuclear staining. (*Courtesy of* Dr Mark Stoler, MD.)

European studies are also emerging to address the utility of dual staining in patients with negative cytology but positive hr-HPV test result (in women older than 30 years). A retrospective analysis by Roelens et al found that dual p16/Ki-67 staining as an adjunct reflex test identified more than 90% of women with underlying HSIL. Reflex testing in this setting reduced colposcopy by one-fourth.[20] These results suggest a role for CINtec+ as a complementary immunocytochemical stain to cytology and hr-HPV testing in selected patient populations.

In addition, the usefulness of dual staining for glandular lesions has been recently evaluated.[31,34] Glandular lesions in cytology can be especially challenging, as they are rare and pathologists tend to err on overdiagnosis, leading to possible overtreatment. Biomarker use, such as dual staining, therefore, represents a unique adjunct marker to cytology and hr-HPV testing. In the largest study to date, Ravarino and colleagues[35] showed that 92.5% of neoplastic samples were positive with CINtec+ and 93.8% of negative samples lacked appropriate dual staining. Noteworthy, the criteria for dual positivity may differ in glandular lesions. The investigators observed that for glandular lesions, morphology and obvious positivity of entire glandular groups was more reproducible than positivity in a single cell.

PRACTICAL APPLICATIONS OF CINTEC+

CINtec+'s niche in cervical cancer screening as a potentially highly sensitive and specific biomarker requires further investigation. It has been noted that the interpretation of CINtec+ with SurePath

(Becton, Dickinson, and Company, Franklin Lakes, NJ) specimens is more difficult than with ThinPrep (ThinPrep Pap test, Hologic, Marlborough, MA), as SurePath-prepared slides contain more crowded and 3-dimensional groups. Complex cell clusters can limit the proposed ease of interpretation of the dual stain.[28]

Large prospective studies are currently under way. As with hybrid capture, a positive immunocytochemical stain does not indicate the type of HPV causing the positive test. Although CINtec+ might serve as a good screening tool, it probably will not be used routinely in addition to hybrid capture techniques.

MINICHROMOSOME MAINTENANCE PROTEIN 2 AND DNA TOPOISOMERASE IIα (PROEX C)

ProEx C (BD Diagnostics, Tripath Imaging Inc, Burlington, NC) is a cocktail of 2 monoclonal antibodies directed at minichromosome maintenance protein 2 (MCM2) and DNA topoisomerase IIα (TOP2A). MCM2 and TOP2A are proteins involved in the regulation of DNA replication during the S-phase of the cell cycle. In the setting of HPV infection, E2F activation leads to aberrant induction of the S-phase, resulting in overexpression of MCM2 and TOP2A.[36,37]

ProEx C is a nuclear stain, which requires the appropriate cytomorphologic features of dysplasia for a positive result (**Fig. 3**). Interpretative pitfalls include staining of normal basal cells, parabasal cells in the setting of atrophy, as well as glandular cells and tubal metaplasia.[9]

Fig. 3. ProExC stain of a squamous cell carcinoma demonstrating the strong nuclear staining (original magnification ×200). (*Courtesy of* Dr Christina Kong, MD.)

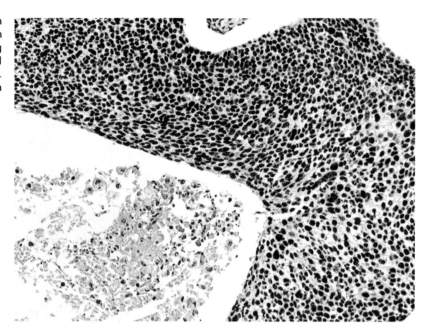

THERAPEUTIC AND PROGNOSTIC APPLICATIONS OF PROEX C

In tissue, several studies have evaluated the utility of ProEx C showing that it is a reliable confirmatory marker for the identification of HSIL. In comparison with other biomarkers, ProEx C is a less sensitive and specific marker than p16 but a more sensitive marker than Ki-67 for the identification of HSIL.[38,39] A combination cocktail of p16 and ProEx C may provide the highest diagnostic value for the detection of HSIL.[38–40] According to the LAST recommendations, insufficient data are currently available to recommend the use of ProEx C as an adjunct biomarker in the evaluation of cervical biopsies.[17]

Regarding cervicovaginal cytology samples, the utility of ProEx C has been assessed in a limited number of studies with the SurePath and the ThinPrep platforms. The biomarker was first studied by Kelly and colleagues[41] and Shroyer and colleagues[42] demonstrating that ProEx C is a reliable immunocytochemical stain increasing the positive predictive value for the detection of HSIL in liquid-based cytology. Halloush and colleagues[21] compared ProEx C with p16 and Ki-67 in cell blocks prepared from residual liquid-based cervicovaginal cytology specimens. They found a comparable performance of ProEx C to p16 and Ki-67. In a larger study by Tambouret and colleagues,[43] ProEx C in conjunction with cytology reached a sensitivity and specificity of 92% and 84%, respectively, for the detection of HSIL. In 2011, Depuydt and colleagues[44] evaluated the efficacy of different cervical cancer screening approaches in 3126 women and concluded that primary hr-HPV screening followed by Pro-Ex C triage represented the best strategy. Most recently, ProEx C has been applied as a distinguishing immunocytochemical stain in the differential diagnosis of hyperchromatic crowded groups.[45]

PRACTICAL APPLICATIONS OF PROEX C

Although ProEx C appears to be a promising biomarker, its specific role in cervical cancer screening requires larger prospective studies and a standardized immunocytochemical processing and scoring protocol. Staining of bacteria and obscuring inflammatory cells, as well as strong background staining, also can make the interpretation of ProEx C challenging.[14]

IN SITU HYBRIDIZATION

In situ hybridization (ISH) for HPV uses a DNA cocktail probe targeting complementary sequences of 13 hr-HPV genotypes, including HPV 16 and 18. If a probe binds to its complementary HPV sequence, a primary dye-specific antibody detects this complex. A secondary biotinylated antibody will subsequently bind, and a chromogenic enzyme (streptavidin-conjugated alkaline phosphatase) produces a colorimetric signal, which can be detected by light microscopy.[46]

ISH is a direct probe method of detecting hr-HPV. It is a slide- based methodology, using residual material from liquid-based cervicovaginal samples or formalin-fixed paraffin-embedded tissue. The analytic sensitivity of ISH for HPV is approximately 10 to 50 viral copies per cell. A diffuse dark navy-blue nuclear signal represents the presence of HPV in episomal form. A blue punctate pattern represents HPV integration into the host DNA (Fig. 4). Signal detection must be correlated with the appropriate cytomorphologic features of the cell. The slide interpretation requires expertise, time, and may be subject to interobserver variability.[47] In addition, artifactual nonspecific staining may be found in neutrophils, eosinophils, nucleoli, and lymphocytes.

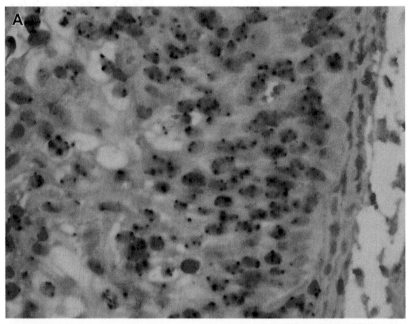

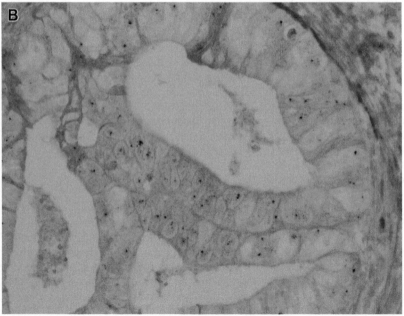

Fig. 4. Positive nuclear staining for in situ hybridization for HPV in a squamous cell carcinoma (*A*, original magnification ×400) and an adenocarcinoma (*B*, original magnification ×400).

Key Points
IMMUNOCYTOCHEMISTRY

- Immunocytochemical stains may represent an alternative approach to HPV triage in women with mild cytologic abnormalities

- The interpretation of p16 and ProEx C requires correlation with the appropriate cytomorphologic features of dysplasia

- The strength of the dual stain lies in its simplicity of interpretation: >1 cell with brown cytoplasmic staining for p16 and red nuclear staining for Ki-67 irrespective of morphology

- Dual staining may be a helpful reflex test for identifying HSIL in women (>30 years of age) with negative Pap test and positive hr-HPV results

Pitfalls
IMMUNOCYTOCHEMISTRY

! p16 can demonstrate false-positive staining (eg, tubal metaplasia, endometrial cells)

! ProEx C can demonstrate false-positive staining (normal basal cells, parabasal cells (atrophy), glandular cells, tubal metaplasia, inflammatory cells and bacteria)

! Dual stain is considered positive only if simultaneous brown cytoplasmic staining for p16 and red nuclear staining for Ki-67 are present

THERAPEUTIC AND PROGNOSTIC APPLICATIONS OF HPV IN SITU HYBRIDIZATION

In contrast to Digene's Hybrid Capture 2 (HC2) (Qiagen, Gaithersburg, MD), no large clinical validation trials have been undertaken to study the utility of ISH in cervical cancer screening. Few smaller studies have compared the performance of ISH to HC2 producing conflicting results. Qureshi and colleagues[48] compared HC2 to ISH for ThinPrep cervical cytology in a prospective study and reported an increased sensitivity without loss of specificity for ISH. A subsequent study for LSIL cytology by Qureshi and colleagues[49] showed a comparable sensitivity and superior specificity to Digene's HC2. These results have

not been confirmed by a second independent group. Hesselink and colleagues[50] reported that ISH lacked the analytical sensitivity in ThinPrep samples to reliably detect HSIL. Davis-Devine and colleagues[51] reported similar findings for SurePath samples in that ISH lacked sensitivity to reliably detect HSIL. These results suggest that ISH may require a more significant infection with HPV to reach adequate detectable levels.

PRACTICAL APPLICATIONS OF IN SITU HYBRIDIZATION

HPV ISH can be extremely useful in tissue sections, especially in differentiating endometrial carcinoma from endocervical carcinoma, and adenocarcinoma in situ versus tubal metaplasia. Its utility in the Pap test is questionable and is not recommended to be used in place of other methods of HPV detection in cervical cytology samples.

Key Points
IN SITU HYBRIDIZATION

- ISH can be helpful in distinguishing endometrial carcinoma invading into the endocervix from endocervical carcinoma

- ISH has not proven to be as effective in identifying hr-HPV in cytologic preparations as alternative methods

HYBRID CAPTURE

Randomized clinical trials, such as the ASC-US Low-Grade Triage Study and Kaiser Permanente Northern California Medical Care Plan, have validated the use of hybrid-capture HPV testing in conjunction with Pap tests and shown that it is more sensitive than cytomorphology alone in detecting high-grade squamous intraepithelial lesions.[52,53] Two methods approved by the Food and Drug Administration (FDA) use hybrid capture: Digene Hybrid Capture 2 High-Risk HPV Test and Cervista HPV High Risk Test (Hologic, Inc, Bedford, MA). Both tests give an assessment of whether hr-HPV is present but do not specify which HPV is the cause of the infection.

Hybrid Capture Diagnostic Assays

Digene HC2
The Digene HC2 assays denature nucleic acids to form single-stranded DNA. Collections

of single-stranded RNA probes corresponding to 13 hr-HPV DNA targets are added to the sample. If the hr-HPV DNA is present in the sample, it will hybridize to the RNA probes. Phosphatase-conjugated antibodies to the RNA:DNA hybrid are coated on microwells and capture the hybrid molecule. Then a chemiluminescent substrate is added and any bound RNA:DNA hybrids cleave the chemiluminescent substrate, which emits a light detectable by a luminometer and is measured as relative light unit. The intensity of the light emitted correlates to the presence or absence of HPV DNA.[54] This threshold value has been determined by the company and validated with large studies.

Cervista HPV high-risk test

The Cervista HPV High Risk Test uses the Invader chemistry to identify specific nucleic acid sequences from 14 hr-HPV types. When probe oligonucleotides specific for DNA targets and an Invader oligonucleotide overlap by at least 1 base pair, a cleavase enzyme cleaves the 5′ portion of the probe at the point of overlap. This 5′ probe piece binds to an added fluorescence resonance energy transfer oligonucleotide, which after a second cleavase enzyme, results in a fluorescence signal. The test comes with positive and negative controls.[54]

THERAPEUTIC AND PROGNOSTIC APPLICATIONS OF HYBRID CAPTURE

Hybrid capture has integrated into current management strategies for screening women for cervical dysplasia and cancer. Only hr-HPV types should be tested, as low-risk types have little impact on management because they are not oncogenic.[55] A stand-alone positive hybrid capture result has a 92% to 96% sensitivity in detecting CIN2+ and a specificity of about 62%.[56,57] This sensitivity is about 14% higher than a repeat Pap test.[57] Currently, cotesting of cytology and HPV is the preferred method of maximizing sensitivity and specificity.

Cotesting of cytology and hybrid capture has a negative predictive value of 0.001.[57] This very low risk of harboring a high-grade lesion allows for safe increase in the screening time interval. The 2012 American Society for Colposcopy and Cervical Pathology (ASCCP) guidelines for the management of abnormal cervical cancer screening tests recommend cotesting with cytology and hr-HPV testing at 5-year increments.[55] Cotesting is not recommended for women younger than 30 due to the high incidence of transient HPV infections in this group. The

current ASCCP guidelines also recommend reflex HPV testing in the setting of a Pap interpretation of ASCs.[55] Hybrid capture reflex testing in young women (21–24 years of age) is acceptable but not preferred, as the incidence of HPV infection is high in this age group. Hence, in this age group, reflex testing would not discern persistent lesions from transient infections well enough to change management.

In a Kaiser study, 4% of women were found to be cytology negative and HPV positive by hybrid capture. Immediate colposcopy did not improve the detection of identifying HSIL significantly enough to warrant this blanket recommendation, so it is suggested to cotest in 1 year in that setting.[55]

Occasionally, there is cross-reaction, with low-risk HPVs resulting in false-positive results. Additionally, too frequent repeated testing reduces the advantage of hybrid capture. Another limitation from a treatment perspective is that hybrid capture results are positive or negative for the presence of hr-HPV, not indicating which hr-HPV subtype is present. The inclusion of HPV types that rarely cause cancer also increases the rate of false-positive results. Therefore, HC alone is good for detecting a high-risk infection but fails to identify a specific hr-HPV subtype or persistence of infection.

PRACTICAL APPLICATIONS OF HYBRID CAPTURE

Hybrid capture has become a common practice in the screening for cervical dysplasia. It aids tremendously in triaging women with an ASC Pap to observation or colposcopy and assists the clinician in localization to endocervix or upper genital tract in women with abnormal glandular cells.[55,58] Both forms of hybrid capture can be used in Cytolyt (Hologic Inc, Bedford, MA) or transport media. However, the media used for liquid-based preparations for SurePath can result in degradation of the HPV DNA and is not FDA-approved for HPV testing.[59] This has become a controversial topic especially in large laboratories that have completed their own clinical validation of using SurePath media. Getting precise numbers is challenging, as there are no false-negative results data published by Becton, Dickinson, but the general issues at hand are as follows:

- SurePath is FDA approved for Pap tests but not for HPV testing.
- If a laboratory choses to use the SurePath collection for hybrid capture then it becomes an off-label use of the test, is considered a

Key Points
Hybrid Capture

- Identification of hr-HPV greatly assists in triaging women with minimal cytologic atypia on Pap tests

- A negative Pap test and hybrid capture test has such a high negative predictive value that screen interval may be safely increased to 5 years

- Two main companies manufacture hybrid capture assays: Digene and Cervista

laboratory-developed test, and requires rigorous laboratory validation.
- Approval for using SurePath for HPV testing was submitted to the FDA several times but each time was withdrawn.
- In June of 2012, the FDA issued a warning to Becton, Dickinson, and Company and then collaboratively issued a bulletin to customers reiterating that SurePath is not FDA-approved for Hybrid Capture 2 and that "Use of the SurePath sample may under certain conditions produce false-negative results…"
- Alternatives to laboratories that wish to maintain the SurePath Pap test include switching buffers or having the clinician co-collect (one for cytomorphology and one in media acceptable for HPV testing).[59–61]

It is important that a hybrid capture test finds the clinically relevant processes. If a test is too sensitive, it will result in a decreased specificity by the overdiagnosis of clinically irrelevant infections.

Pitfalls
Hybrid Capture

! Cross reactivity with low-risk HPV and inclusion of hr-HPV types that rarely cause cancer can result in false-positive results

! Hybrid capture does not identify the specific genotype of HPV causing the infection

! A laboratory must perform its own validation of methods if it decides to use an HPV test that is not FDA certified or different from the manufacturer's protocol

This issue arose with Cervista HPV testing. Some researchers found that Cervista test positivity was 2 to 4 times more positive than other tests.[62] Being set at too high of a sensitivity, the test resulted in too many women getting unnecessary colposcopies.[62] Overall, the limiting factor for hybrid capture is that it does not identify which hr-HPV is causing the infection and that it cannot distinguish transient from persistent hr-HPV infections. This is where genotyping plays a role.

GENOTYPING

Because most squamous cell carcinomas are the result of HPV 16 or 18 infections, and the identification of these 2 genotypes is associated with a higher probability of progressing to a high-grade lesion, great attention has recently been given to genotyping for HPV 16 and 18.[9] Genotyping allows for type-specific HPV detection, which can then influence management decisions.

GENOTYPING DIAGNOSTIC ASSAYS

Genotyping assays approved by the FDA include APTIMA 16/18/45 Genotype Assay (GenProbe, San Diego, CA) and Cobas HPV test (Roche Molecular Systems, Pleasanton, CA). The Hologic Cervista HPV 16/18 test uses the same Invader chemistry described previously for hybrid capture. However, the probe oligonucleotides bind specifically to the DNA sequences of HPV 16 and 18.

The APTIMA detects E6/E7 mRNA transcripts from 14 hr-HPV types but does not isolate individual infections. It shows high sensitivity and specificity and has little to no cross-reactivity to low-risk HPV types. However, a second genotype assay, the APTIMA 16/18/45, can be performed that discriminates HPV 16 and HPV 18/45 (it does not separate HPV 18 from HPV 45). The process consists of 3 steps: target capture, amplification by transcription-mediated amplification (TMA), and detection of the amplification products by the Hybridization Protection Assay.[63]

The Cobas HPV test uses polymerase chain reaction to amplify target DNA sequences. It then uses nucleic acid hybridization for a single analysis in the detection of 14 hr-HPV types and specifically identifies HPV 16 and 18.[64,65]

The ATHENA trial (Addressing THE Need for Advanced HPV diagnostics) was a US multicenter (61 centers) trial developed to assess whether the addition of genotyping aided in risk stratification of women having CIN 2 or greater, and whether HPV 16 or 18 genotyping could assist in management decisions.[63] The study found that detecting HPV 16 and HPV 18 predicted the presence of CIN 3 or greater with 92.0% sensitivity and 56.9% specificity. Cotesting with cytology increased the sensitivity by less than 5% but resulted in a 30% increase in screen positives.[66] This trial suggests that genotyping alone may be a viable alternative to Pap test with reflexive genotyping.

THERAPEUTIC AND PROGNOSTIC APPLICATIONS OF GENOTYPING

It is currently FDA-approved to use genotyping in the setting of ASCUS diagnoses and in screening patients 30 years of age or older. Women with positive hr-HPV DNA can have HPV 16 or 18 genotyping performed to better stratify management. The 2012 Consensus Guidelines for the Management of Women with Abnormal Cervical Cancer Screening Tests recommended that women with HPV 16 or 18 positivity should be referred for colposcopy, whereas those with negative HPV 16 or 18 can be rescreened in 1 year either by cytology or repeat HPV testing.[55] Some studies have found that when compared with hybrid capture, genotyping is less sensitive but more specific for identifying CIN2+.[63] The negative predictive value of genotyping and cytology is 99.7%.[6]

An additional finding of the ATHENA trial is the utility of genotyping in different age populations. The prevalence of hr-HPV in an ASCUS setting varies with age (65% in 22–28-year-olds vs 19.5% in woman older than 40).[58] Additionally, the incidence of having a high-grade lesion on biopsy is reduced in the older population.[63] Adding genotyping allows a clinician to react more conservatively if the lesion in not secondary to HPV 16 or HPV 18.

PRACTICAL APPLICATIONS AND CHALLENGES OF GENOTYPING

Many of these genotyping tests have been validated through large, multi-institutional studies. The current recommended approach for using genotyping is in women with negative cytology and positive hr-HPV with hybrid capture.[1,55] However, stand-alone HPV DNA testing is proving to be an equally viable screening method. This topic becomes extremely important for a laboratory considering bringing on HPV tests that are not FDA-approved, as they necessitate the laboratory independently validating the assays being considered. It is often difficult for a single laboratory to have the volume or controlled end points for the validation. Moreover, the cost of molecular testing may present an obstacle to its benefits.

Key Points
GENOTYPING

- Genotyping allows for specific identification of HPV 16 and HPV 18 infections and better assessment of persistence of an infection
- Genotyping assays approved by the FDA include APTIMA 16/18/45 Genotype Assay and Cobas HPV test and the Hologic Cervista HPV 16/18
- A laboratory must validate any genotyping test that is not FDA approved
- Achieving the numbers and outcome points equivalent to the multicenter trial can be challenging

FUTURE TRENDS

Cervical cancer screening is changing at a rapid clip. As we better understand the biology of HPV, we have seen a shift in the screening strategy. Screening is now initiated at an older age (21 in the United States, 25 or older in many other countries), and screening intervals are expanding. Although in the United States the vast majority of women still get Pap tests first, additional methods are being used to further screen for HPV types. As molecular tests become more common and easier to implement within a laboratory, we may also see a shift away from cytomorphology as a primary means for screening. With the advent of large studies validating methods and the vaccination of young women to the most aggressive hr-HPV types, it may be that morphology tests drop precipitously and the identification of hr-HPV by hybrid capture followed by genotyping or genotyping alone becomes the front line of screening. Although not accepted in the United States yet, many European countries have moved to HPV screening as the first means of triage for women.[67]

REFERENCES

1. Agorastos T, Sotiriadis A, Chatzigeorgiou K. Can HPV testing replace the Pap test? Ann N Y Acad Sci 2010;1205:51–6.
2. Doorbar J, Quint W, Banks L, et al. The biology and life-cycle of human papillomaviruses. Vaccine 2012;30(Suppl 5):F55–70.
3. Saslow D, Solomon D, Lawson HW, et al. American Cancer Society, American Society for Colposcopy and Cervical Pathology, and American Society for

Clinical Pathology screening guidelines for the prevention and early detection of cervical cancer. Am J Clin Pathol 2012;137(4):516–42.

4. Sherman M, Abdul-Karin F, Berek J, et al. Chapter 4. Atypical squamous cells. In: Solomon D, Nayar R, editors. The Bethesda system for reporting cervical cytology. 2nd edition. New York: Springer; 2004. p. 67–87.

5. Pitman M, Cibas E, Pwers C, et al. Reducing or eliminating use of the category of atypical squamous cells of undetermined significance decreases the diagnostic accuracy of the Papanicolaou smear. Cancer 2002;96(3):128–34.

6. Davey D, Greenspan D, Kurtycz D, et al. Atypical squamous cells, cannot exclude high-grade squamous intraepithelial lesion: review of ancillary testing modalities and implications for follow-up. J Low Genit Tract Dis 2010;14(3):206–14.

7. Galgano M, Castle P, Stoler M, et al. Can HPV-16 genotyping provide a benchmark for cervical biopsy specimen interpretation? Am J Clin Pathol 2008;130(1):65–70.

8. Gupta N, Srinivasan R, Rajwanshi A. Functional biomarkers in cervical precancer: an overview. Diagn Cytopathol 2010;38(8):618–23.

9. Pinto A, Degen M, Villa L, et al. Immunomarker in gynecologic cytology: the search for the ideal "biomolecular Papanicolaou test". Acta Cytol 2012;56: 109–21.

10. Dray M, Russell P, Dalrymple C, et al. p16INK4a as a complementary marker of high-grade intraepithelial lesions of the uterine cervix. I: Experience with squamous lesions in 189 consecutive cervical biopsies. Pathology 2005;37(2):112–24.

11. Stoler MH. Toward objective quality assurance: the eyes don't have it. Am J Clin Pathol 2002;117: 520–2.

12. Pantanowitz L, Florence RR, Goulart RA, et al. *Trichomonas vaginalis* P16 immunoreactivity in cervicovaginal Pap tests: a diagnostic pitfall. Diagn Cytopathol 2005;33(3):210–3.

13. Mulvany NJ, Allen DG, Wilson SM. Diagnostic utility of p16 INK4a: a reappraisal of its use in cervical biopsies. Pathology 2008;40(4):335–44.

14. Oberg T, Kipp B, Vrana J, et al. Comaprison of p16INK4a and ProEx C immunostaining on cervical ThinPrep cytology and biopsy specimens. Diagn Cytopathol 2010;38:564–72.

15. Klaes R, Benner A, Friedrich T, et al. p16INK4a immunohistochemistry improves interobserver agreement in the diagnosis of cervical intraepithelial neoplasia. Am J Surg Pathol 2002;26(11): 1389–99.

16. Galgano MT, Castle PE, Atkins KA, et al. Using biomarkers as objective standards in the diagnosis of cervical biopsies. Am J Surg Pathol 2010;34(8): 1077–87.

17. Darragh TM, Colgan TJ, Thomas Cox J, et al. The Lower Anogenital Squamous Terminology Standardization project for HPV-associated lesions: background and consensus recommendations from the College of American Pathologists and the American Society for Colposcopy and Cervical Pathology. Int J Gynecol Pathol 2013;32(1): 76–115.

18. Tsoumpou I, Arbyn M, Kyrgiou M, et al. p16INK4a immunostaining in cytological and histological specimens from the uterine cervix: a systematic review and meta-analysis. Cancer Treat Rev 2009;35: 210–20.

19. Denton KJ, Bergeron C, Klement P, et al. The sensitivity and specificity of p16INK4a cytology vs. HPV testing for detecting high-grade cervical disease in the triage of ASCUS and LSIL Pap cytology results. Am J Clin Pathol 2010;134:12–21.

20. Roelens J, Reuschenbach M, Von Knebel Doeberitz M, et al. p16INK4a immunocytochemistry versus human papillomavirus testing for triage of women with minor cytologic abnormalities. A systematic review and meta-analysis. Cancer Cytopathol 2012;120:294–307.

21. Halloush R, Akpolat I, Zhai Q, et al. Comparison of ProEx with p16INK4a and Ki-67 immunohistochemical staining of cell blocks prepared from residual liquid based cervicovaginal material. Cancer Cytopathol 2008;114(6):474–80.

22. Beccati MD, Buriani C, Pedriali M, et al. Quantitative detection of molecular markers ProEx C (minichromosome maintenance protein 2 and topoisomerase IIa) and MIB-1 in liquid-based cervical squamous cell cytology. Cancer 2008;114: 196–203.

23. Yu L, Wang L, Zhong J, et al. Diagnostic value of p16INK4A, Ki-67, and human papillomavirus L1 capsid protein immunochemical staining on cell blocks from residual liquid-based gynecologic cytology specimens. Cancer Cytopathol 2010; 118:47–55.

24. Sahebali S, Depuydt CE, Segers K, et al. Ki-67 immunocytochemistry in liquid based cervical cytology: useful as an adjunctive tool? J Clin Pathol 2003;56:681–6.

25. Schmidt D, Bergeron C, Denton K, et al. p16/Ki-67 dual-stain cytology in the triage of ASCUS and LSIL papanicolaou cytology. Results from the European Equivocal or Mildly Abnormal Papanicolaou Cytology Study. Cancer Cytopathol 2011;119(3): 158–66.

26. Atkins K. p16/Ki67 dual-stain cytology in the triage of ASCUS and LSIL papanicolaou cytology. Cancer Cytopathol 2011;119(3):145–7.

27. Samarawardana P, Singh M, Shroyer KR. Dual stain immunohistochemical localization of p16INK4A and ki-67: a synergistic approach to

identify clinically significant cervical mucosal lesions. Appl Immunohistochem Mol Morphol 2011; 19(6):514–8.

28. Edgerton N, Cohen C, Siddiqui M. Evaluation of CINtec PLUS testing as an adjunctive test in ASC-US Diagnosed Surepath Preparations. Diagn Cytopathol 2011;41(1):35–40.

29. Chivukula M, Austin M, Matsko J, et al. Use of dual-stain for p16 and Ki67 in the interpretation of abnormal Pap cytology results: a prospective study (abstract). Cancer Cytopathol 2010;118(Suppl 5): 333–4.

30. Loghavi S, Walts AE, Bose S. CINtec® plus dual immunostain: a triage tool for cervical pap smears with atypical squamous cells of undetermined significance and low grade squamous intraepithelial lesion. Diagn Cytopathol 2012. http://dx.doi.org/10.1002/dc.22900.

31. Donà MG, Vocaturo A, Giuliani M, et al. p16/Ki-67 dual staining in cervico-vaginal cytology: correlation with histology, human papillomavirus detection and genotyping in women undergoing colposcopy. Gynecol Oncol 2012;126(2):98–202.

32. Singh M, Mockler D, Akalin A, et al. Immunocytochemical colocalization ofP16(INK4a) and Ki-67 predicts CIN2/3 and AIS/adenocarcinoma. Cancer Cytopathol 2012;120(1):26–34.

33. Waldstrøm M, Christensen RK, Ørnskov D. Evaluation of p16(INK4a)/Ki-67 dual stain in comparison with an mRNA human papillomavirus test on liquid-based cytology samples with low-grade squamous intraepithelial lesion. Cancer Cytopathol 2013;121(3):136–45.

34. Meyer JL, Hanlon DW, Andersen BT, et al. Evaluation of p16INK4a expression in ThinPrep cervical specimens with the CINtec p16INK4a assay: correlation with biopsy follow-up results. Cancer 2007; 111(2):83–92.

35. Ravarino A, Nemolato S, Macciocu E, et al. CINtec PLUS immunocytochemistry as a tool for the cytologic diagnosis of glandular lesions of the cervix uteri. Am J Clin Pathol 2012;138(5):652–6.

36. Malinowski D. Multiple biomarkers in molecular oncology: I. Molecular diagnostics applications in cervical cancer detection. Expert Rev Mol Diagn 2007;7:117–31.

37. Santin AD, Zhan F, Bignotti E, et al. Gene expression profiles of primary HPV 16- and HPV 18-infected early stage cervical cancers and normal cervical epithelium: identification of novel candidate biomarkers for cervical cancer diagnosis and therapy. Virology 2005;331:269–91.

38. Shi J, Liu H, Wilkerson M, et al. Evaluation of p16INK4a, minichromosome maintenance protein 2, DNA topoisomerase IIalpha, ProEx C, and p16INK4a/ProEx C in cervical squamous intraepithelial lesions. Hum Pathol 2007;38:1335–44.

39. Badr R, Walts A, Chung F, et al. BD ProEx C: a sensitive and specific marker of HPV-associated squamous lesions of the cervix. Am J Surg Pathol 2008; 32(6):899–905.

40. Pinto AP, Schlecht NF, Woo TY, et al. Biomarker (ProEx C, p16(INK4A), and MiB-1) distinction of high-grade squamous intraepithelial lesion from its mimics. Mod Pathol 2008;21(9):1067–74.

41. Kelly D, Kincaid E, Fansler Z, et al. Detection of cervical high-grade squamous intraepithelial lesions from cytologic samples using a novel immunocytochemical assay (ProExTMC). Cancer 2006;108: 494–500.

42. Shroyer K, Homer P, Heinz D, et al. Validation of a novel immunocytochemical assay for topoisomerase IIa and minichromosome maintenance protein 2 expression in cervical cytology. Cancer 2006; 108:324–30.

43. Tambouret RH, Misdraji J, Wilbur DC. Longitudinal clinical evaluation of a novel antibody cocktail for detection of high-grade squamous intraepithelial lesions on cervical cytology specimens. Arch Pathol Lab Med 2008;132(6):918–25.

44. Depuydt CE, Makar AP, Ruymbeke MJ, et al. BD-ProExC as adjunct molecular marker for improved detection of CIN2+ after HPV primary screening. Cancer Epidemiol Biomarkers Prev 2011;20(4): 628–37.

45. Ge Y, Mody DR, Smith D, et al. p16(INK4a) and ProEx C immunostains facilitate differential diagnosis of hyperchromatic crowded groups in liquid-based Papanicolaou tests with menstrual contamination. Acta Cytol 2012;56(1):55–61.

46. Gustafson KS, Clark DP. Molecular cytopathology. In: Tubbs RR, Stoler MH, editors. Cell and tissue based molecular pathology. 1st edition. Philadelphia: Churchill Livingstone Elsevier; 2009. p. 173–4.

47. Hubbard RA. Human papillomavirus testing methods. Arch Pathol Lab Med 2003;127:940–5.

48. Qureshi MN, Rudelli RD, Tubbs RR, et al. Role of HPV DNA testing in predicting cervical intraepithelial lesions: comparison of HC HPV and ISH HPV. Diagn Cytopathol 2003;29(3):149–55.

49. Qureshi MN, Bolick D, Ringer PJ, et al. HPV testing in liquid cytology specimens: comparison of analytical sensitivity and specificity for in situ hybridization and chemiluminescent nucleic acid testing. Acta Cytol 2005;49(2):1–9.

50. Hesselink AT, van den Brule AJ, Brink AA, et al. Comparison of hybrid capture 2 with in situ hybridization for the detection of high-risk human papillomavirus in liquid-based cervical samples. Cancer 2004;102(1):11–8.

51. Davis-Devine S, Day SJ, Freund GG. Test performance comparison of inform HPV and hybrid capture 2 high-risk HPV DNA tests using the SurePath

liquid-based Pap test as the collection method. Am J Clin Pathol 2005;124(1):24–30.

52. Stoler M. Testing for human papillomavirus: data driven implications for cervical neoplasia management. Clin Lab Med 2003;23(3):569–83.

53. Rebolj M, Bonde J, Njor SH, et al. Human papillomavirus testing in primary cervical screening and the cut-off level for hybrid capture 2 tests: systematic review. BMJ 2011;342:d2757.

54. Arbefeville S, Bossler A. Chapter 33. Human papillomavirus. In: Schrijver I, editor. Diagnostic molecular pathology in practice. Berlin: Springer-Verlag; 2011. p. 269–75.

55. Massad L, Einstein M, Huh W, et al. 2012 updated consensus guidelines for the management of abnormal cervical cancer screening tests and cancer precursors. Obstet Gynecol 2013;121(4):829–46.

56. Castle PE, Solomon D, Wheeler CM, et al. Human papillomavirus genotype specificity of hybrid capture 2. J Clin Microbiol 2008;46:2595–604.

57. Arbyn M, Sasieni P, Merjer C, et al. Clinical applications of HPV testing: a summary of meta-analysis. Vaccine 2006;24(3):S78–89.

58. Katki H, Schiffman M, Castle P, et al. Five-year risks of CIN 3+ and cervical cancer among women with HPV-positive and HPV-negative high-grade Pap results. J Low Genit Tract Dis 2013;17(5 Suppl 1):S50–5.

59. Castle P. A response to an article in USA Today. Available at: http://rubbermeetstheroad.me/a-response-to-an-article-in-usa-today/. Accessed September 18, 2013.

60. Zhao C, Yang H. Approved assays for detecting HPV DNA, design indications, and validation. Northfield (IL): CAP Today; 2012.

61. Ortega B. False-negative results found in HPV testing. Pheonix (AZ): The Arizona Republic; 2013.

62. Kinney W, Stoler M, Castle P. Special commentary: patient safety and the next generation of HPV DNA tests. Am J Clin Pathol 2010;134(2):193–9.

63. Sherman ME, Schiffman M, Cox T. Effects of age and human papilloma viral load on colposcopy triage: data from the randomized Atypical Squamous Cells of Undetermined Significance/Low-Grade Squamous Intraepithelial Lesion Triage Study (ALTS). J Natl Cancer Inst 2002;94:102–7.

64. Heideman DA, Hesselink AT, Berkhof J, et al. Clinical validation of the cobas 4800 HPV test for cervical screening purposes. J Clin Microbiol 2011;49:3983–5.

65. Stoler M, Wright T, Sharma A, et al. Evaluation of HPV 16 and HPV 18 genotyping for the triage of women with high risk HPV+ cytology negative results. Am J Clin Pathol 2011;135:468–75.

66. Castle P, Stoler M, Wright T, et al. Performance of carcinogenic HPV testing and HPV 16 or HPV 18 genotyping for cervical cancer screening of women aged 25 years and older; a subanalysis of the ATHENA study. Lancet Oncol 2011;12:880–90.

67. Giorgi R, Ronco G. The present and future of cervical cancer screening programmes in Europe. Curr Pharm Des 2013;19(8):1490–7.

Metastatic Tumors of Unknown Origin

Ancillary Testing in Cytologic Specimens

Sara E. Monaco, MD*, David J. Dabbs, MD

KEYWORDS

- Metastasis • Unknown primary • Fine-needle aspiration • Cytopathology • Molecular • Testing
- Cytology

ABSTRACT

The application of ancillary studies, such as immunostains, to cytopathology has improved the ability to make accurate diagnoses with precise subclassification. Even with these techniques, there are still aspiration and exfoliative cytology cases for which it remains difficult to definitively determine the source and/or subtype. This article focuses on the well-established and novel ancillary studies used in the modern era of cancer diagnoses in cytopathology, particularly in the diagnostic work-up of metastatic tumors without a known primary.

OVERVIEW

Cancer of unknown primary includes a heterogeneous group of metastatic tumors that have no definitive primary tumors or origin. These tumors of unknown primary are thought to represent approximately 3% to 5% of all solid organ malignancies and are usually associated with a dismal prognosis.[1,2] These cases present unique challenges in that there is no site-directed therapy that can be offered without knowing the origin of a tumor, which usually leads to broad-spectrum empiric chemotherapy that can be ineffective. Determining the exact origin of a tumor can benefit patients by making them eligible for certain site-specific therapies and thereby improve their quality of life and prognosis. Thus, characterization of these tumors is of great interest to patients and oncologists and has become a rapidly evolving area as more and more novel biomarkers and tests are created.[3,4]

A majority of tumors of unknown origin are adenocarcinomas, followed by squamous cell carcinomas and neuroendocrine carcinomas, and are detected in the liver, bone, or brain at a late stage.[5,6] Although a majority of these tumors have a poor prognosis, approximately 20% have a better prognosis, including germ cell tumors and lymphomas. The tumors that most often present without an identifiable primary lesion include adenocarcinomas arising from the lung or pancreatobiliary or gastrointestinal tract and melanoma.[6] Some of these tumors, in particular malignant melanoma cases without a known primary, may be attributed to a primary that was simply missed on examination or a lesion that was previously removed without a diagnosis or could be due to immune-induced regression of the primary lesion.[7] In a study looking at spinal

Conflict of Interest Statement: The authors have no financial or personal relationships with other people or organizations that could inappropriately influence (bias) the content of this article.

Department of Pathology, Magee Women's Hospital, University of Pittsburgh Medical Center, 300 Halket Street, Pittsburgh, PA 15213, USA

* Corresponding author. Department of Pathology, University of Pittsburgh Medical Center, 5150 Centre Avenue, POB2, Suite 201, Pittsburgh, PA 15232.

E-mail address: monacose@upmc.edu

Surgical Pathology 7 (2014) 105–129

http://dx.doi.org/10.1016/j.path.2013.10.004

metastases, 13% had no known primary and a majority of these were adenocarcinomas.[8] In an autopsy study, clinically occult primaries were identified in 75% of patients with carcinomas of unknown primary, and approximately 50% of these tumors were found to have pulmonary, pancreatic, or gastrointestinal origin.[9] There are also approximately 8% of patients with carcinomas of unknown primary who have a latent primary, which is a primary that is clinically identified after the initial diagnosis of carcinoma of unknown primary.[10] In most cases, the type of tumor can be determined based on a combination of cytomorphologic features in conjunction with clinicoradiologic findings and ancillary test results, including immunocytochemistry (ICC), in situ hybridization, and gene expression profiling.

CYTOMORPHOLOGIC ASSESSMENT

Patients with a tumor of unknown origin usually present with multiple solid organ lesions (eg, liver, bone, brain, or lung masses), lymphadenopathy, and/or peritoneal carcinomatosis, depending on the type of tumor. Thus, these tumors can be encountered in aspiration or exfoliative cytology specimens, and the tumors may be of epithelial origin (eg, carcinoma) or nonepithelial origin (eg, lymphoma, melanoma, sarcoma, and mesothelioma). In general, fine-needle aspiration (FNA) biopsies and other cytologic specimens offer a minimally invasive diagnostic modality with a sensitivity of approximately 60% to 95% and specificity close to 100%.[11] False-negative diagnoses, largely due to sampling error, compromise the sensitivity in cytologic specimens. The advent of superior imaging techniques may be able to increase the sensitivity, in addition to the use of rapid on-site evaluation, which can maximize the sensitivity and diagnostic yield of FNA and minimize the nondiagnostic rate. Body fluid cytology is also commonly used to evaluate patients with tumors of unknown primary because the specimen is easy to acquire through minimally invasive methods (eg, thoracentesis). Exfoliative cytology specimens differ from aspiration cytology, however, in that there are many normal cells in the background (eg, mesothelial cells and histiocytes), whereas aspiration specimens are typically enriched with tumor cells. This is especially important in interpreting the results of immunostains and molecular studies, in that there must be certainty in characterizing the tumor cells of interest as opposed to the normal background cells (**Fig. 1**).

Fig. 1. Metastatic adeno-carcinoma of colorectal origin in peritoneal fluid. This fluid specimen shows cohesive clusters of tumor cells in a background of reactive mesothelial cells, lymphocytes, and histio-cytes. (*A*) The cell block highlights the columnar nature of the tumor cells, nuclear pleomorphism, and prominent nucleoli. (*A*) Diff-Quik stain, orig-inal magnification ×400; (*B*) hematoxylin-eosin stain, original magnifi-cation ×400.

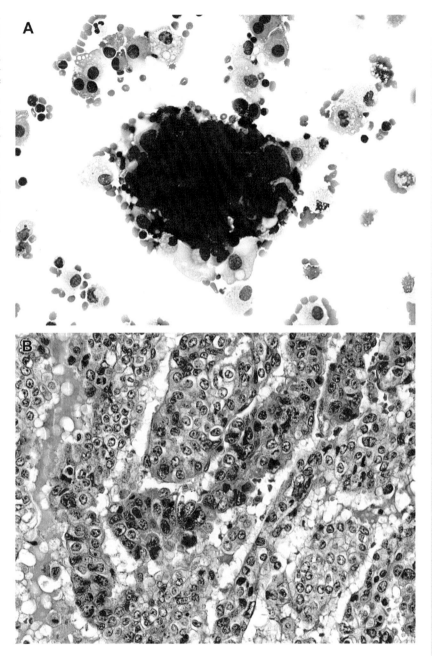

The initial cytomorphologic evaluation is impor-tant in these cases to determine which studies are needed and to help allocate the appropriate material for these necessary and confirmatory ancillary studies. Some of the key tumor types with their corresponding key morphologic features and defining ancillary study results are listed in Table 1 (Fig. 2). In general, cohesion is usually a

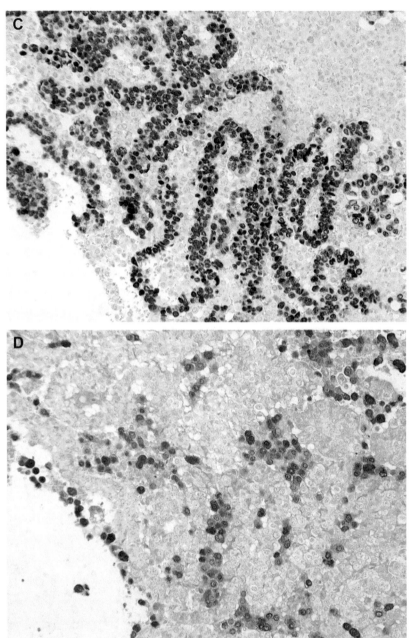

Fig. 1. (continued). Metastatic adenocarcinoma of colorectal origin in peritoneal fluid. Immunostains performed on the cell block showed that the tumor cells are positive for CDX2 (C), in addition to CK20 and MOC31. The tumor cells showed negative staining for calretinin (D), and WT-1, which highlight the background mesothelial cells. (C, D) immunostains, original magnification ×400.

trademark of carcinomas and mesotheliomas, whereas discohesion is usually a feature of melanoma, sarcoma, and lymphoma. In carcinomas, vacuolated cytoplasm, prominent nucleoli, and mucin production are features of an adenocarcinoma, whereas dense cytoplasm, intercellular bridges, and keratinization have been used to identify a squamous cell carcinoma. Some studies

Table 1
Differential diagnosis for tumor of unknown origin in cytopathology specimens and applicable ancillary studies

Tumor Type	Basic Cytomorphology	ICC Panel	Molecular Studies and Other
Adenocarcinoma	Cohesive, vacuolated cytoplasm, prominent nucleoli	MOC31, BerEP4, B72.3/TAG, CK, site-specific markers (eg, TTF-1, CDX2)	Molecular studies for theranostic information (eg, lung [*EGFR, KRAS, BRAF, ALK*], colon [*BRAF* and *KRAS*])
Squamous cell carcinoma	Cohesive, dense cytoplasm, coarse chromatin, orangeophilia on Papanicolaou stain	p40/p63, CK5/6, site-specific markers (p16, HPV)	HPV CISH
Lymphoma	Discohesive, lymphoglandular bodies	CD45, CD20, CD3, subtype-specific markers (eg, CD30, ALK, EBV)	FC and FISH studies for clonality (eg, IGH rearrangement or T-cell gene rearrangement) and subtyping (eg, specific immunophenotype by FC or specific translocation by FISH)
Melanoma	Discohesive, binucleation, prominent nucleoli, intranuclear inclusions, melanin pigment	S-100, melan-A, HMB45, tyrosinase, MiTF	Molecular studies for theranostic information (eg, *BRAF* and *KRAS*)
Sarcoma	Discohesive, marked nuclear pleomorphism, scant to moderate amounts of cytoplasm	Vimentin, subtype-specific markers (eg, desmin)	FISH studies for subtyping (eg, *EWS* translocations)
Mesothelioma	Cohesive with spaces between cells, nucleoli, two-tone cytoplasm	WT-1, calretinin, D2–40, CK5/6, cytokeratin, GLUT1	FISH for diagnostic and prognostic information (eg, *p16* deletion by FISH)

Abbreviation: FC, flow cytometry.

have shown that cytology is superior to histology in subclassification due to the use of multiple stains, including the Papanicolaou stain, which allows for better cellular detail and accentuates keratinization in squamous cell carcinomas.[12,13] This may account for the lower dependence on immunoperoxidase stains in cytology than in small biopsies due to the superior morphologic detail, particularly in the diagnosis of squamous cell carcinoma.[13] Morphologic features can also help in determining the source of an unknown tumor, such as columnar tumor cells in an inflammatory and necrotic background from a metastatic colonic adenocarcinoma (see **Fig. 1**) or pigmented pleomorphic single cells from a metastatic malignant melanoma (see **Fig. 2**B). The tumor type and origin may not be clear, however, based on the cytomophology, even with immunostains and other ancillary studies. In addition, cytology specimens may lack sufficient material for evaluation, necessitating additional work-up.

ANCILLARY STUDIES IN DIAGNOSIS

The goal of ancillary studies is to hone in on the specific type of tumor (eg, lymphoma vs carcinoma vs sarcoma) and the origin of the tumor (eg, lung, gastrointestinal, or breast), which may not be possible by morphologic examination alone. For this reason, allocating material for ancillary studies is crucial in these cases.

IMMUNOCYTOCHEMISTRY

ICC has become the most commonly used ancillary diagnostic study applied to cytologic specimens. This is partly because cytologic diagnoses supported by immunostains have higher interobserver agreement and more-specific diagnoses and minimize the chance of having a tumor that cannot be further classified.[14,15] For instance, in respiratory cytology, cytomorphologic evaluation alone results in accurate subclassification of pulmonary non–small cell carcinomas in approximately 60% of cases (66% for adenocarcinoma and 53% for squamous cell carcinomas),[16] whereas the use of immunostains has reduced the rate of unclassifiable lung tumors to less than 7% and increased the accuracy of the cytologic diagnosis.[15] Thus, in most cases, particularly poorly differentiated non–small cell carcinomas, the use of an immunopanel or special stains for

Fig. 2. Cytomorphology of main types of tumors, other than adenocarcinoma, that could be responsible for a tumor of unknown origin. (*A*) Metastatic renal cell carcinoma shows prominent clustering, with prominent nucleoli and vacuolated cytoplasm. (*B*) Metastatic malignant melanoma is characterized by discohesion with binucleation, prominent nucleoli, intranuclear inclusions, and occasionally cytoplasmic melanin pigment. (*A, B*) Diff-Quik stain, original magnification ×400.

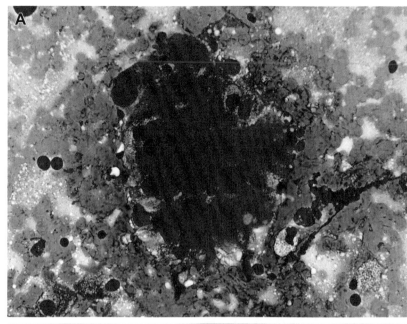

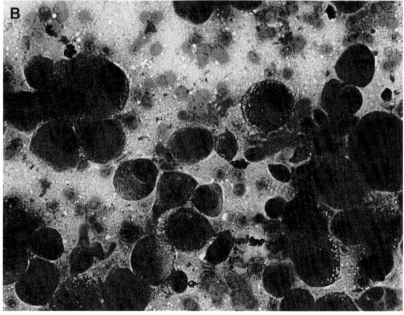

adenocarcinoma (eg, thyroid transcription factor 1 [TTF-1], Napsin A, cytokeratin [CK]7, and mucicarmine) and squamous cell carcinoma (eg, p40, p63, CK5/6, and glypican 3) has become standard practice.[14,17] In general, the combination of cytomorphology, clinical information, and ICC predicts the origin of a tumor in approximately 40% to 70% of cases.[6,10]

An initial panel of immunostains commonly used in the work-up of a metastatic poorly differentiated neoplasm, to determine the cell type or origin, includes pan-CK for epithelial tumors, leukocyte common antigen (LCA/CD45) for lymphomas, S-100 for melanoma, vimentin for sarcoma, and calretinin for mesotheliomas (see **Table 1**). Once the cell of origin is determined, additional

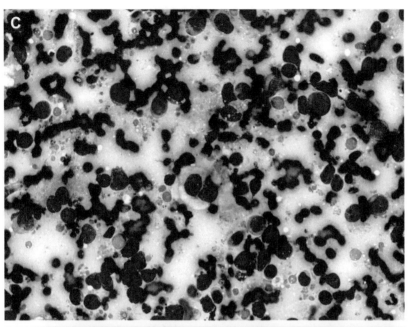

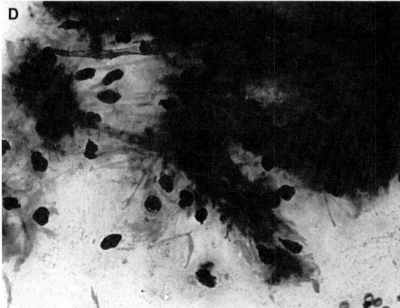

Fig. 2. (continued). Cytomorphology of main types of tumors, other than adenocarcinoma, that could be responsible for a tumor of unknown origin. (C) Lymphoma shows a predominantly discohesive population of cells with a background of lymphoglandular bodies. (D) Sarcomas or mesenchymal neoplasms tend to be discohesive with round to oval nuclei and pleomorphism and may have background fibrous or myxoid material. (C, D) Diff-Quik stain, original magnification ×400.

more-specific markers for each type can be used. For example, in the setting of epithelial tumors, the coordinate expression of cytokeratins 7 and 20 (Table 2), in addition to coexpression of vimentin and site-specific markers (eg, CDX2 and TTF-1) can help determine the tissue of origin (Table 3).[18]

A majority of lung, breast, gastric, and ovarian adenocarcinomas show a CK7-positive/CK20-negative immunophenotype. In fluid cytology, however, other markers of mesothelial cells should also be included in the panel, given that mesothelial cells stain positive for CK7 and could mimic

Table 2
Differential diagnosis for carcinoma of unknown primary based on CK7/CK20 profile

CK7+/CK20+	CK7+CK20−	CK7−/CK20+	CK7−/CK20−
Urothelial	Lung	Gastrointestinal	Squamous cell carcinoma
Pancreatobiliary	Breast	Merkel cell carcinoma	Adrenal
Upper gastrointestinal	Thyroid	Small cell carcinoma of the salivary gland	Liver (hepatocellular carcinoma)
Ovary (mucinous)	Salivary gland	—	Renal (clear cell)
—	Pancreatobiliary	—	Prostate
—	Upper gastrointestinal	—	Lung (small cell carcinoma)
—	Female genital tract (endometrial, endometrioid tumors, serous tumors, nonmucinous ovarian)	—	Nonepithelial tumors (lymphoma, sarcoma)
—	Mesothelial	—	Thymus
—	Renal cell carcinoma (papillary and chromophobe)	—	—
—	Squamous cell carcinoma of cervix	—	—

Table 3
Site-specific markers for carcinoma of unknown primary

Tumor Origin	Site-Specific Immunostains[a]
Lung	TTF-1, Napsin A
Gastrointestinal	CDX2, CK20
Breast	Mammaglobin, GCDFP15, ER, PR
Ovary	PAX8, WT1
Pancreatobiliary	CA19-9
Thyroid	Thyroglobulin, TTF-1, PAX8
Prostate	PSA, PSAP, NKX3.1
Urothelial	GATA3, uroplakin 3
Renal	PAX8, RCC, CD10
Germ cell	PLAP, OCT3/4
Squamous cell carcinoma from head and neck, uterine cervix, or anogenital	p16

Abbreviations: CA, carbohydrate antigen; PLAP, placental alkaline phosphatase; PSA, prostate-specific antigen; PSAP, prostate-specific alkaline phosphatase; RCC, renal cell carcinoma; WT, Wilms tumor.

[a] Note: No immunostain is entirely specific as a site-specific marker; however, these stains tend to be associated with these tumor origins with a relatively high specificity.

a CK7-positive metastatic adenocarcinoma. TTF-1 can also be added as a highly sensitive and specific marker in differentiating pulmonary adenocarcinomas from other CK7-positive tumors. The CK7-negative/CK20-positive and CDX2-positive immunoprofile is highly specific for an adenocarcinoma of colorectal origin, although a few gastric and pancreatic adenocarcinomas exhibit this immunoprofile as well (see **Fig. 1**).[19] Vimentin expression with CK can be seen with tumors of endometrial, thyroid, renal, salivary gland or mesothelial origin. More site-specific markers are being developed and validated given their usefulness in the setting of a tumor of unknown primary (see **Table 3**). For instance, in the setting of lung adenocarcinoma, Napsin A has been introduced to help in difficult cases and is positive in more than 80% of lung adenocarcinoma, with a higher specificity than TTF-1.[20] Thus, cytoplasmic positivity of Napsin A can be supportive evidence of an adenocarcinoma of lung and is particularly helpful in cases of equivocal TTF-1 staining because only rare nonpulmonary adenocarcinomas report as Napsin A positive (eg, renal cell carcinoma).[17] Although most site-specific markers do not determine the site of origin for a squamous cell carcinoma, immunostaining for p16 or in situ hybridization for HPV can be helpful in cases of metastatic squamous cell carcinoma of unknown primary, because these stains could help confirm an

HPV-related squamous cell carcinoma arising from the oropharynx, anogenital region, or uterine cervix (**Fig. 3**).[21,22] ICC is particularly helpful in those tumors that are poorly differentiated and show only subtle features of an adenocarcinoma or squamous cell carcinoma, in that immunostains have been shown to refine these tumors into a particular subtype in 65% to 75% cases.[14–16] Thus, ICC plays an instrumental role in being able to determine the tumor type and site of origin for tumors of unknown primary. For this reason, acquiring sufficient material for cell block is of utmost importance in modern cytopathology so that there are tumor cells available for these crucial studies.

> ### Key Points
> #### TUMORS WITH COEXPRESSION OF CYTOKERATIN AND VIMENTIN
>
> - Endometrial adenocarcinoma
> - Renal cell carcinoma
> - Salivary gland carcinoma
> - Spindle cell carcinoma or sarcomatoid carcinoma
> - Thyroid carcinoma
> - Mesothelioma
> - Uncommon in tumors arising from endocervix, gastrointestinal tract, breast, lung, and prostate

Nonepithelial tumors can present as tumors of unknown primary and should be suspected in tumors that fail to show CK staining or have cytomorphologic features suggesting a nonepithelial tumor (eg, discohesion). These tumors include malignant melanoma, lymphoma, sarcoma, germ cell tumor, and some pediatric malignant small round blue cell tumors (see **Fig. 2**). Malignant melanoma is immunoreactive for HMB45, S-100, melan-A, tyrosinase, and other melanoma markers. Perivascular epithelioid tumors and neurogenic tumors (eg, malignant peripheral nerve sheath tumors) can also show S-100 positivity. CK immunoreactivity is rarely seen in malignant melanoma and sarcoma and should not be seen in lymphomas. Sarcomas account for only 3% to 6% of malignant effusions and rarely present as a tumor of unknown origin. Synovial sarcoma, epithelioid sarcoma, vascular tumors, leiomyosarcoma, endometrial stromal sarcoma, and gastrointestinal stromal tumor (GIST) are some of the

sarcomas that can present as tumors of unknown origin. Although vimentin is positive in sarcomas, it can also be positive in a subset of carcinomas (eg, renal and endometrial), mesotheliomas, and lymphomas. In children, the most common causes of a tumor of unknown primary are the small round blue cell tumors, such as lymphoma and leukemia, followed by Wilms tumor, neuroblastoma, Ewing sarcoma, and rhabdomyosarcomas. In these scenarios, flow cytometry and ICC play an important role.

> ### Key Points
> #### UTILITY OF IMMUNOCYTOCHEMISTRY IN THE DIAGNOSIS OF TUMORS OF UNKNOWN PRIMARY
>
> - Important for tumors without distinctive morphologic differentiation.
> - Enhances the ability to make an accurate and specific diagnosis.
> - Helpful to determine the cell of origin (eg, epithelial, lymphoma, sarcoma, or melanoma).
> - Site-specific markers can identify the site of origin (eg, TTF-1 and CDX2).
> - Can predict the site of origin in approximately 40% to 70% of cases.
> - Reduces the proportion of unclassifiable lung tumors to less than 7%.

Furthermore, there must be awareness of the limitations of immunostains in cytology specimens, including the need for a sufficient number of cells to characterize, quality control, and the appropriate processing.[23,24] Obtaining enough cells to characterize can be a challenge in bloody or hypocellular specimens. Thus, additional passes dedicated for cell block or an additional thin core biopsy can be beneficial. Material can also be preserved by cutting additional unstained slides upfront with the initial hematoxylin-eosin–stained slide to avoid the loss of tissue with trimming of the block. Quality control with the appropriate positive and negative controls is also of utmost importance when dealing with immunostains. This is particularly important to ensure that the stain is working when there is negative staining in the specimen and to make sure there is no artifactual staining. False-negative results can occur due to sampling issues when the tumor cells are not well represented on the cell block. False-positive results can occur with nonspecific

Fig. 3. Metastatic squamous cell carcinoma of tonsillar origin. Squamous cell carcinoma showing nuclear pleomorphism, coarse chromatin, and dense cytoplasm. (*A*) Diff-Quik stain, original magnification ×400; (*B*) hematoxylin-eosin stain, original magnification ×400.

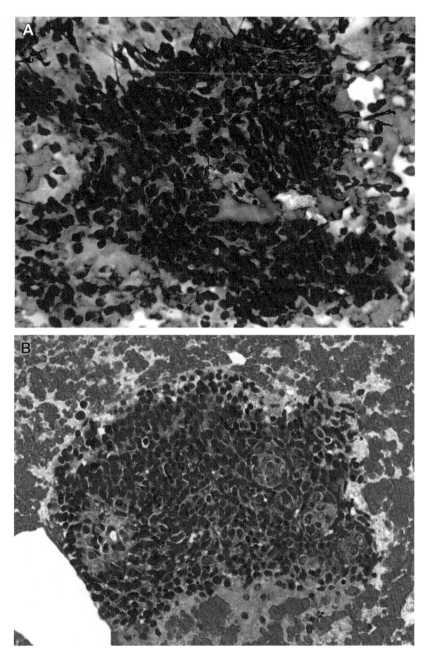

staining or high background. The processing of the specimen can also matter, particularly with antibodies that are labile or difficult. One example is with alcohol fixatives, which can decrease the staining with certain antibodies, including S-100, HepPar1, and ER.[24,25] A critical item to remember is that although ICC plays an important role in the diagnosis of metastatic tumors of unknown origin,

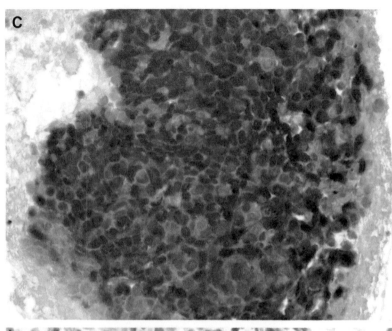

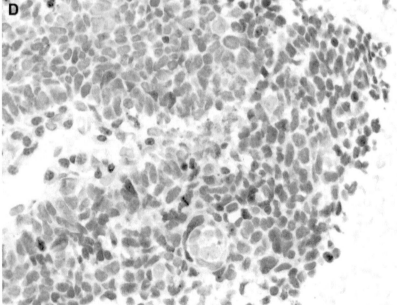

Fig. 3. (*continued*). Metastatic squamous cell carcinoma of tonsillar origin. Squamous cell carcinoma showing nuclear pleomorphism, coarse chromatin, and dense cytoplasm. Diffuse, strong positivity for p16 by ICC (*C*) and dot-like positivity for HPV by CISH (*D*) can help in establishing a diagnosis of an HPV-related squamous cell carcinoma of the head and neck, uterine cervix, or anogenital region. (*C*) p16 immunostain, original magnification ×400; and (*D*) CISH for HPV, original magnification ×400.

the findings must be correlated with the morphology. It is well known that many immunostains tend to be very sensitive but not very specific. For example, when dealing with small round blue cell tumors, CD99 is not only expressed in Ewing sarcoma but also has been seen in lymphoblastic lymphomas, poorly differentiated synovial sarcoma (including the round cell variant), Merkel cell carcinoma, desmoplastic small round cell tumors, and other tumors. Furthermore, even with optimal fixation, quality control, and sufficient cellularity, not every tumor can be successfully subclassified by ICC.

Pitfalls
DIAGNOSTIC PITFALLS OF IMMUNOCYTOCHEMISTRY IN THE DIAGNOSIS OF TUMORS OF UNKNOWN PRIMARY

! ICC requires sufficient viable tumor cells for analysis.

! ICC needs appropriate fixation and processing (eg, cell block preparation for an immunopanel).

! Alcohol fixatives can decrease staining with some antibodies (eg, S-100, HepPar1, and ER).

! Quality control is essential to make sure antibodies are working appropriately.

! Correlation with morphology is important given nonspecific staining with certain antibodies.

! False-negative results may be due to sampling error, interpretation error, or inappropriate fixation.

! False-positive results may be due to interpretation error or overstaining.

IN SITU HYBRIDIZATION

FISH probes target specific chromosomal regions of interest to detect gene rearrangements or translocations, deletions, and gene amplifications, which are helpful to confirm clonality in hematolymphoid malignancies and to subtype malignancies (**Table 4**). FISH can be performed on fixed tissue, and cytology specimens are ideal given that they provide whole cells with no nuclear truncation, which allows more accurate signal counting. Also, decalcified bone surgical specimens may not be suitable for FISH, whereas aspirates from bone do not need to be decalcified and are superior for testing. In a lymphoid neoplasm, if flow cytometry is indeterminate or unavailable, then FISH studies can be done on the fixed cells to look for an IGH or T-cell receptor gene rearrangement to confirm clonality. In addition, specific translocations, like the t(8;14) translocation seen in Burkitt lymphoma and the t(11;14) translocation seen in mantle cell lymphoma, can help subclassify a lymphoma. Similarly, FISH studies in sarcomas can also help with precise subtyping.

The best example is a small round blue cell tumor, where *EWS* gene rearrangements could be detected by FISH to support a diagnosis of Ewing sarcoma, and other gene rearrangements can also be performed to exclude other entities, such as the *FOXO1* translocation in alveolar rhabdomyosarcomas and the t(X;18) translocation in synovial sarcoma. FISH studies are also emerging as a helpful study in salivary gland tumors, because new translocations are discovered in different subtypes of salivary gland tumors, including the *ETV6-NTRK3* gene fusion in mammary analog secretory carcinoma and the *MECT1-MAML2* translocations in mucoepidermoid carcinomas. Cytogenetics and FISH studies can also assist in diagnosing new variants of renal cell carcinoma with specific genetic abnormalities that are now recognized by the latest World Health Organization (WHO) classification. This includes renal cell carcinoma with the Xp11.2/*TFE3* gene translocations, typically seen in young women. FISH studies can also help confirm malignancy in mesothelial proliferations, which can be challenging because morphology alone cannot always distinguish benign from malignant mesothelial cells. In these scenarios, FISH studies for the *p16* gene deletion can help in that this deletion is seen primarily in mesotheliomas and seems absent in reactive mesothelial proliferations.[26]

Key Points
UTILITY OF FISH IN THE DIAGNOSIS OF TUMORS OF UNKNOWN PRIMARY

• FISH detects genetic abnormalities associated with certain tumors (eg, translocations, deletions, and amplifications).

• FISH can be performed on fixed cells (eg, no fresh specimen required).

• Cytology specimens are superior to decalcified bone specimens.

• Aspirate smears provide whole nuclei to avoid nuclear truncation artifacts seen with tissue sections.

• FISH can confirm a clonal hematolymphoid population.

• FISH can subtype lymphoid tumors, sarcomas, salivary gland tumors (eg, mammary analog secretory carcinoma), and renal tumors (eg, renal cell carcinoma with the Xp11.2/*TFE3* gene translocations).

• FISH can detect genetic abnormalities that correlate with treatment or prognosis.

Unlike ICC, which is universally available, FISH studies require more technical expertise and results have a longer turnaround time. In addition, FISH cannot detect all chromosomal abnormalities that are detectable with classical genetics and cannot be performed on specimens processed with certain fixatives, such as eosin, harsh acids, and decalcification solutions.

post-transplant lymphoproliferative disorders (PTLDs). CISH can be done on paraffin-embedded cell block material and has the same challenges seen with FISH, including the requirement for appropriate facilities and expertise and slower turnaround time than ICC.

Pitfalls

DIAGNOSTIC CHALLENGES IN FISH STUDIES PERFORMED ON CYTOLOGY SAMPLES OF TUMORS OF UNKNOWN PRIMARY

! FISH cannot detect other chromosomal abnormalities that are detected with classical cytogenetics.

! FISH requires technical expertise.

! FISH may not be amenable to specimens processed with certain fixatives (eg, eosin, harsh acids, and decalcification).

! Results take longer turnaround time than ICC (approximately 3 days).

Key Points

UTILITY OF CISH IN THE DIAGNOSIS OF TUMORS OF UNKNOWN PRIMARY

• Diagnosis of certain lymphomas that have a well-established link to EBV (eg, EBV-positive diffuse large B-cell lymphoma of the elderly and PTLD)

• Confirming origin of a squamous cell carcinoma of unknown origin (eg, HPV-related head and neck [eg, tonsil], uterine cervix, or anogenital squamous cell carcinoma)

Key Points

DIFFERENTIAL DIAGNOSIS OF HPV-RELATED SQUAMOUS CELL CARCINOMAS

• Oropharyngeal, including tonsil

• Uterine cervix

• Anogenital

CISH is also emerging as a helpful test in the diagnosis of tumors of unknown primary, particularly in squamous cell carcinomas. The association of HPV with squamous cell carcinomas occurring in the head and neck region (eg, tonsil), uterine cervix, and anogenital area has led to the utility of detecting HPV in metastatic squamous cell carcinomas to help determine the site of origin (see **Fig. 3**).[21,22] This is particularly helpful in the setting of lung tumors with squamous morphology, in patients with a history of an HPV-related squamous cell carcinoma, or in metastatic squamous cell carcinomas to a neck lymph node with no known primary. Traditionally, the origin of a squamous cell carcinoma has been unable to be determined due to lack of site-specific ICC markers that stain these tumors. The positivity for p16 by ICC, however, which is a surrogate marker for HPV, and the use of CISH for detection of HPV have enabled determining if a metastatic squamous cell carcinoma represents a metastasis from a new undetected primary in the head and neck, cervix, or anus. CISH also is important in lymphomas to prove an association with Epstein-Barr virus (EBV), particularly for new subtypes recognized by the WHO classification that depend on the detection of HPV, such as EBV-positive diffuse large B-cell lymphoma of the elderly and

MOLECULAR PROFILING

In recent years, molecular profiling of tumors has become increasingly popular to determine the origin of tumors with an unknown primary based on conventional methods (ie, morphology and immunoprofile). These studies initially involved oligonucleotide microarrays, which tend to be complex and time consuming. Thus, there was a shift to primarily using mRNA and microRNA in polymerase chain reaction (PCR) assays and gene expression microarrays to screen for genes of interest in classification and treatment (**Table 5**).[4] The usefulness of these tests is that they help guide oncologists toward more site-specific therapies that may have better efficacy in these patients. In addition, newer assays, like next-generation sequencing, can identify potential mutations that are amenable to targeted therapies, as opposed to precise determination of the tissue of origin, and likely is of greater

Table 4
Key diagnostic FISH studies for tumor of unknown origin

Tumor Type	Specific Diagnosis	Diagnostic FISH Study
Hematolymphoid	Follicular lymphoma	t(14;18): IGH-bcl2
	Diffuse large B-cell lymphoma	t(14;18)(q32;q21): IGH and bcl2 (30%)
		bcl-6, bcl-2, and c-myc gene
		rearrangements
	Mantle cell lymphoma	t(11;14): bcl-1/cyclin D1-IGH
	Burkitt lymphoma	t(8;14): c-myc and IGH (75%)
		t(2;8): Ig kappa and c-myc (15%)
		t(8;22): c-myc and Ig lambda (10%)
	Marginal zone lymphoma (MALT	Trisomy 18
	lymphomas)	Trisomy 3
		t(11;18): API2 and MLT
	Chronic lymphocytic leukemia/small	Deletion 13q14
	lymphocytic lymphoma	Deletion 11q23
		Trisomy 12
	Anaplastic large cell lymphoma	t(2;5): ALK and NPM
Epithelial (carcinoma)	Mammary analog secretory carcinoma	t(12;15): ETV6-NTRK3 fusion gene
	Mucoepidermoid carcinoma	t(11;19): MECT1-MAML2
	Renal cell carcinoma associated with Xp11.2/TFE3 gene fusions	Xp11.2 rearrangements
	Undifferentiated midline carcinoma	t(15;19): NUT-BRD4 fusion
	Thymic carcinoma	
Germ cell tumor	Seminoma	Isochromosome 12p
Mesenchymal (sarcoma)	Alveolar soft part sarcoma	t(X;17): ASPL-TFE3 fusion gene
	Extraskeletal myxoid chondrosarcoma	t(9;22): CHN-EWS fusion gene
	Clear cell sarcoma	t(12;22): ATF1-EWSR1 fusion gene
	Congenital/infantile fibrosarcoma	t(12;15): ETV6-NTRK3 fusion gene
	Mesoblastic nephroma	
	Desmoplastic small round cell tumor	t(11;22): WT1-EWS fusion gene
		t(21;22): ERG-EWS fusion gene
	Ewing sarcoma/PNET, extraosseous	t(11;22): FLI1-EWS fusion gene
		t(21;22): ERG-EWS fusion gene
		t(2;22): FEV-EWS fusion gene
		t(7;22): ETV1-EWS fusion gene
		t(17;22): E1AF-EWS fusion gene
	Inflammatory myofibroblastic tumor	Translocations at 2p23 involving ALK gene
	Myxoid liposarcoma	t(12;16): TLS-CHOP/FUS fusion gene or
		t(12;22): CHOP-EWS fusion gene
	Well-differentiated liposarcoma	Marker ring or giant chromosome 12q13–15
		Amplification of MDM2 and CDK4
	Low-grade fibromyxoid sarcoma	t(7;16): FUS-CREB3L2
		t(11;16): FUS-CREB3L1
	Alveolar rhabdomyosarcoma	t(2;13): PAX3-FKHR
		t(1;13): PAX7-FKHR
	Synovial sarcoma	t(X;18): SYT-SSX fusion

Abbreviations: Ig, immunoglobulin; MALT, mucosa-associated lymphoid tissue; PNET, primitive neuroectodermal tumor.

importance as more genes and targeted therapies are discovered.[2,4,6,27] The advantages need to be weighed against the disadvantages, however, which include the high cost of these molecular tests and the inability to characterize all tumors. A comparison of the advantages and disadvantages in the two most commonly used tests for tumors of unknown origin, ICC and molecular genetic profiling, is in **Table 6**.

Molecular profiling of tumors of unknown primary has been performed in a few different assays and shown feasible with an accuracy of

Table 5
Molecular assays for determining tumor origin by gene expression profiling

Assay Company and Test Name	Type of RNA	FDA Approved	Type of Tissue Preferred	Application to Cytology
Agendia (CupPrint) Amsterdam, Netherlands www.agendia.com	mRNA	No	Frozen or FFPE tissue (average tumor content of 65%)[34]	Possible (no specific studies on cytology specimens)
bioTheranostics (CancerTYPE ID) San Diego, California www.biotheranostics.com	mRNA	No	FFPE tissue (300–500 viable tumor cells needed or 40% tumor cells with minimal necrosis and <6 y old)[35]	Yes, FNA and fluid cell blocks acceptable (10% cases studied included FNA cell blocks but excluded fluid cell blocks)[35]
Pathwork Diagnostics (Tissue of Origin Test)[a] Redwood City, California www.pathworkdx.com	mRNA	Yes	FFPE tissue (greater than or equal to 60% non-necrotic tumor and <8 y old)[29]	Yes, FNA and fluid cell blocks acceptable (studied in body fluids and FNAs)[29]
Rosetta Genomics (ProOncTumorSourceDx/ miRview mets) Philadelphia, Pennsylvania www.rosettagenomics.com	miRNA	No	FFPE tissue (tumor cell content of at least 50%)[36]	Yes, FNA and bronchial wash/brush (may be superior for archival tissue)

Abbreviation: FFPE, formalin-fixed, paraffin-embedded.
[a] Pathwork Tissue of Origin Test, at the time of this publication, is no longer offered (see text).

approximately 85% in most studies.[3,5,10,28–34] The 4 major assays are listed in **Table 5**, and most of these assays require high-quality mRNA that can be extracted from most formalin-fixed, paraffin-embedded cell blocks (see **Table 5**). Because of the degradation in mRNA over time, however, archival cell blocks may not have sufficient mRNA, and these older samples may benefit from miRNA analysis, which is available in the Rosetta assay (Rosetta Genomics, Philadelphia, Pennsylvania).[34] In general, these tests compare the gene expression profile in the unknown tumor to a defined gene set to find the closest match. Of these assays, the Pathwork Tissue of Origin Test (Pathwork Diagnostics, Redwood City, California) is the only one currently FDA approved and the one that has been studied most extensively in cytology specimens; recently, however, Pathwork Diagnostics was reported out of business and the Tissue of Origin Test reportedly (at the time of this publication) unavailable.[28] Thus, the future availability of this test is uncertain. CancerTYPE ID (bio-Theranostics, San Diego, California) is an assay using reverse transcriptase–PCR on formalin-fixed, paraffin-embedded tissue and was able to successfully analyze approximately 70% of specimens in a small series.[10] The failed cases were attributed to scant tumor cellularity or poorly preserved RNA. In addition, 75% of the predictions made by the assay were correct based on follow-up data where the molecular results matched the latent primary detected 9 to 314 weeks after the initial diagnosis of carcinoma of unknown primary. The remainder of the cases were incorrect (15%) or unclassifiable (10%) by the molecular profiling. The most common primary sites that were correctly identified included breast, ovary/primary peritoneal, non–small cell carcinomas of the lung, and gastrointestinal tumors. The incorrect predictions included a molecular signature predicting gastrointestinal carcinoma, testicular cancer, and sarcoma in patients with gastric, pancreatic, and lung primaries, respectively. This study excluded FNA biopsy specimens; thus, it is uncertain how small biopsies and cytology specimens will perform with this molecular assay. Small needle core biopsies, however, comprised a third of cases tested with the CUP molecular assay (Veridex, La Jolla, California) and 61% of all cases had a putative tissue origin assigned by the assay.[3] Furthermore, in the subgroup of patients with extensive immunostains performed, the percent of cases of a specific tumor of origin assigned increased from 11% with

Table 6
Comparison of advantages and disadvantages of conventional immunocytochemistry and new gene expression profiling

	Immunocytochemistry	Gene Expression Profiling
Sensitivity	Moderate sensitivity	Moderate to high sensitivity depending on tumor type
Cost	Lower cost	Higher cost
Availablility	Widespread expertise available for performing and interpreting stains	Limited expertise in the performance and interpretation of results
Type of specimen	Requires less cells and applicable to variety of specimens (eg, cytospins, smears, cell block), morphology helps to distinguish tumor cells vs benign cells	Requires sufficient high-quality RNA (eg, cell block or fresh frozen specimen), approximately 30 μg of RNA with at least 40%–60% tumor cells with <20% necrosis
Type of result	Qualitative (±) or semiquantitative	Quantitative
Correlation with cytomorphology	Directly compare morphology and staining pattern	Not directly possible
Use in rare tumors	Limited by lack of reliable site-specific markers for some tumors (eg, pancreatobiliary)	May detect tumors that do not have site-specific ICC markers
Able to characterize all specimens	No	No
Use in archival cell blocks	Possible	May not be possible due to RNA degradation over time
Limitations	• Limited by antibodies available in a laboratory • Need enough tumor cells for multiple slides to perform an extensive panel of stains	• Limited by genes and tumors in particular assay and training set • Genetic profile of tumors are not always homogeneous, causing overlap with other tumor types • Decreased accuracy in poorly differentiated tumors

immunostains alone to 62% with the CUP assay.[29] Cell blocks from body fluid specimens with greater than 60% tumor cellularity were tested with the Pathwork Tissue of Origin Test and 94% of the cases were in agreement with the available diagnosis, which suggests that cytologic material is acceptable for these assays.[28]

Some of the challenges that arise with molecular profiling are related to specimen issues and interpretation issues (see **Table 6**). The issues related to the specimen include the need to have an optimally prepared, sufficient amount of viable tumor cells to have accurate results. This entails microscopic evaluation by a pathologist to confirm that the cells present are viable tumor cells and that there are a sufficient number of the cells to make the test results meaningful. Without this information, a negative result from a molecular test performed on a nonviable tumor sample or a sample of normal tissue may represent a false-negative result and convey the wrong information to the treating physician. For instance, in one study looking at the use of gene expression profiling in metastatic carcinomas of unknown primary in body fluid cytology, one discordant result was seen where the gene expression analysis result supported an ovarian origin in a male patient and, when correlated with the morphology, the specimen was found to have a predominance of mesothelial cells.[28] In addition, in body fluid cases of low tumor cellularity (<60% tumor cellularity), the Pathwork Tissue of Origin Test frequently generated a result indicative of lymphoma, which is likely due to the predominance of small lymphocytes in these effusion specimens.[28] These findings underscore the importance of meticulous specimen selection with high tumor cellularity (>60% viable cells) and minimal background inflammation or benign cells, in addition to correlation with morphology and, ultimately, the clinicoradiologic findings. Furthermore, the specimen needs to be optimally prepared. For example, some tissue blocks are decalcified or fixed in media (eg, Bouin solution) that may not be conducive to most molecular studies. Thus, sending these specimens for testing may involve wasted time and money with the end result unreliable. Overall, it is estimated that approximately 15% of tissue blocks do not have enough tissue available after immunostains and other tests are performed and another 15% fail due to inadequate RNA.[29] The use of cytology specimens and small biopsies needs to be investigated more because these are the types of specimens frequently used for the documentation of metastatic disease, and only a few studies have looked at genetic profiling in these small specimens.[28]

On the interpretation side, the analysis of the molecular results requires a skilled data set to generate a reference database with which to compare individual test results. Furthermore, the genes or proteins investigated need to be biomarkers that have some significance in terms of determining the origin of a tumor or be associated with some prognostic or predictive information that benefit patients and alter their treatment in a meaningful way. Without this, it is a waste of resources and health care dollars to perform tests that have no clinical utility. Furthermore, these tests have to be able to classify cases better than traditional cheaper methods (eg, morphology and ICC), because if these novel molecular assays are indeterminate in cases indeterminate by ICC and only definitive in cases definitive by ICC, then there is probably little utility for doing this more costly test.[35] In addition, the cost difference is important, because the typical 7 to 10 immunostains performed on most cases is far cheaper than the $3500 cost of the tissue of origin test by Pathwork Diagnostics.[5] For this reason, reimbursement of these tests by insurance companies and the Centers for Medicare and Medicaid Services may cease if the findings do not affect health outcomes in a meaningful way. Over time, these issues may be minimized as more standardized algorithms and less expensive platforms arise. As with any ancillary study, the results also need to be correlated with the clinical and radiologic picture and cannot be used in isolation.

Key Points
MOLECULAR GENETIC PROFILING IN THE DIAGNOSIS OF TUMORS OF UNKNOWN PRIMARY

- Novel method for determining the origin of tumors unclassifiable by other tests

- Compares the gene profile in tumor cells to the genes associated with a variety of different tumors in order to find a similar profile

- Identification of a primary tumor could offer better site-directed therapy

- May identify genetic abnormalities associated with predictive or prognostic value

Pitfalls
DIAGNOSTIC CHALLENGES OF MOLECULAR GENETIC PROFILING

! Requires sufficient material in the appropriate fixative/media for testing.

! Needs viable tumor cells for analysis to avoid a false-negative result.

! Requires high-quality nucleic acids for testing without significant degradation.

! Enriched tumor sample is optimal to avoid misinterpretation of benign background cells.

! Correlation with clinicoradiologic information is essential.

! Optimized controls and data sets are critical for the results to be meaningful and accurate.

THERAPEUTIC AND PROGNOSTIC APPLICATIONS

Ancillary studies not only help in diagnosing tumors of unknown origin and elucidating a primary site but also are increasingly used to look for the expression of predictive biomarkers that can help in treatment selection for patients and prognostic markers. This has increased with the expanding array of targeted therapies that give patients better survival and response, in addition to being more tolerable than traditional chemotherapeutic options. Some of these examples include the use of Imatinib (STI-571; Gleevec) for GISTs, trastuzumab (Herceptin) for HER2/neu-positive breast cancers, and rituximab for CD20-positive lymphomas. ICC plays an important role, because immunostains for immunostains for CD117 (c-kit), CD20, Her2/neu, estrogen receptor and progesterone receptor (ER/PR) are routinely evaluated for treatment purposes in GISTs, lymphomas, and breast carcinomas, respectively (**Fig. 4**). Furthermore, molecular studies for mutational analysis and gene translocations in solid organ tumors, such as lung non–small cell carcinomas, are increasing. Next-generation sequencing is also emerging as a way to detect rare mutations that may have targeted therapies available and with this, the focus may change from identifying a primary origin to simply identifying genes of therapeutic significance.

This molecular revolution has been most evident in thoracic cytopathology, moving from a dichotomous classification of lung cancer (eg, small cell vs non–small cell carcinoma) to refining classification of non–small cell carcinomas into squamous cell carcinoma, adenocarcinoma, large cell carcinoma, and other subtypes to determine who could potentially benefit from certain molecular tests and targeted therapies. In addition, there is now an emphasis on maximizing tissue for *EGFR* and *KRAS* mutational studies in addition to FISH studies for *ALK* gene rearrangements to select lung cancer patients who will benefit from tyrosine kinase inhibitor therapy (eg, *EGFR* sensitivity mutations), patients who will not respond and likely have poor prognosis (eg. *KRAS* mutations), and patients who will benefit from crizotinib (eg, *ALK* rearrangement). Other examples of prognostic studies that can be done include FISH studies to detect the presence of a *c-myc* rearrangement in diffuse large B-cell lymphomas that tend to behave more than aggressively. In addition, the presence of a *p16* gene deletion in mesothelioma is also associated with a worse survival for patients.[36] Thus, although, the traditional cytomorphologic assessment is important, these important ICC, molecular, and FISH studies provide important information to guide treatment and prognosis.

Given the importance of these studies, there has been a recent trend to limit the number of ICC stains performed in an effort to maximize the cells available for other studies with predictive or prognostic information. For example, most carcinomas of unknown primary have between 6 and 10 immunostains performed for characterization.[5,26] There is now a paradigm, however, particularly in lung cancer diagnoses, to limit immunostains to smaller panels or to use a staged approach in an effort to limit those cases of exhaustive immunostains and maximize the tissue remaining for potential molecular studies.[14,15,17] In addition, recent studies have used dual staining, which allows for

two immunostains to be performed on the same slide, thereby minimizing tissue even further.[37] In some cases without definitive morphologic differentiation or atypical staining patterns, however, a more extensive panel may be unavoidable and justifiable for precise and accurate subclassification.

> ### *Key Points*
> #### THERAPEUTIC AND PROGNOSTIC STUDIES IN TUMORS OF UNKNOWN ORIGIN
>
> - Biomarkers can be predictive markers to indicate who may respond to targeted therapies.
> - Biomarkers can be prognostic markers.
> - ICC is helpful to evaluate for CD117 in GISTs, CD20 in lymphomas, and HER2/neu or hormone receptor (ER/PR) status in breast carcinomas.
> - Mutational analysis for *EGFR, KRAS, BRAF,* and other common genetic abnormalities is important to select patients for treatment with tyrosine kinase inhibitors.
> - FISH studies for *ALK* gene rearrangements can help select patients for treatment with crizotinib.
> - FISH detection of the *p16* deletion in mesotheliomas is an important negative prognostic marker.

PRACTICAL APPLICATIONS

Ancillary studies have enhanced the ability to subclassify tumors of unknown origin, and new biomarkers are entering daily practice to improve patient care in this era of personalized medicine. In most routine cases, malignancies are evaluated with clinical-radiologic assessment and morphologic analysis to create a preliminary differential diagnosis (**Fig. 5**). In the histology laboratory, cell blocks from cytology specimens necessitating ICC and potential molecular studies should have unstained slides ordered at the time of accessioning to avoid the loss of tissue that occurs when a block is trimmed upon orders added later. These blank slides can then be numbered so that the high-priority tests are done on the slides with more material. Then targeted ICC and molecular studies can be performed depending on the type of tumor. ICC is done in most cases to confirm cell type and tumor origin and this is sufficient in a majority of cases for diagnosis (**Fig. 6**). In general, for a poorly differentiated tumor of unknown

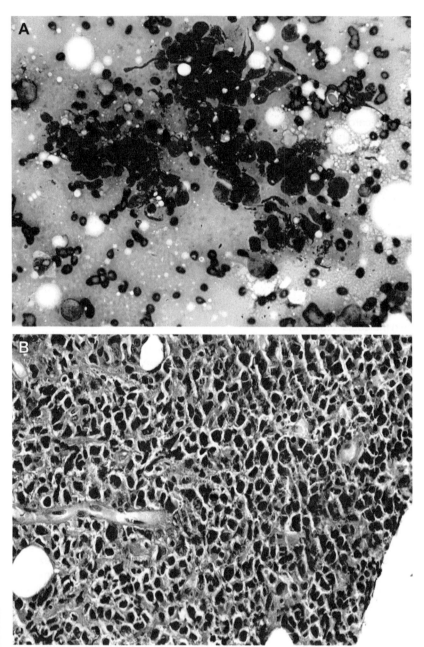

Fig. 4. Malignant diffuse large B-cell lymphoma with CD20-positivity. This lymphoma shows loosely cohesive large tumor cells with prominent nucleoli and crush artifact. (*A*) Diff-Quik stain, original magnification ×400; (*B*) hematoxylin-eosin stain, original magnification ×400.

origin, a pan-CK, CD45 (leukocyte common antigen), S-100, and vimentin stain can help determine the cell type (epithelial, lymphoid, melanoma, or other). Then, for carcinomas, a combination of CK7 and CK20 and site-specific markers can help pinpoint a tissue origin. In cases with an ICC profile that is not entirely specific or with clinical and radiologic findings that are inconclusive, molecular genetic profiling tests may be used to determine the tumor origin. All these tests require sufficient, viable tumor cells for analysis, however, and due to the sampling issues in cytology, not

Fig. 4. (continued). Malignant diffuse large B-cell lymphoma with CD20-positivity. This lymphoma shows loosely cohesive large tumor cells with prominent nucleoli and crush artifact. Due to the clustering, this tumor was thought to be an adenocarcinoma; however, ICC revealed this was a CD20-positive (C) B-cell lymphoma. The CD3 stain (D) highlights a few background T-cells but is negative in the larger tumor cells of interest. (C, D) immunostains, original magnification ×400.

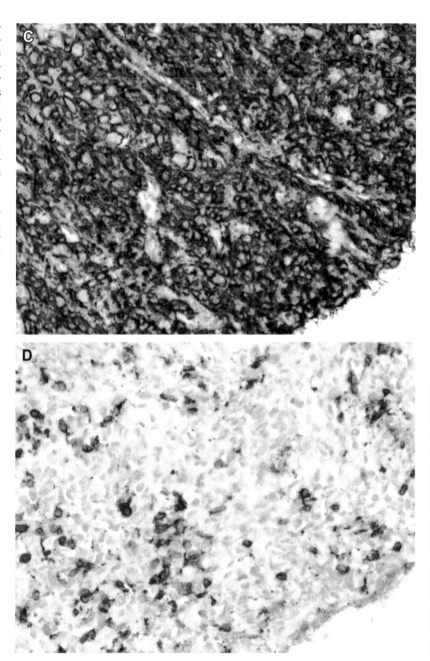

every tumor may be amenable to definitive subtyping. Thus, it is critical to not order a multitude of unnecessary tests upfront but to do so in a staged manner to preserve tissue and avoid the need for larger tissue biopsies or excisions. Overall, the improvement of ICC stains with an expanding array of antibodies for a variety of tumors, including some antibodies of therapeutic importance, in addition to the advent of gene expression profiling assays, has improved the ability to define the origin of certain tumors, which, in turn, may lead to better site-specific treatments.[1] As more

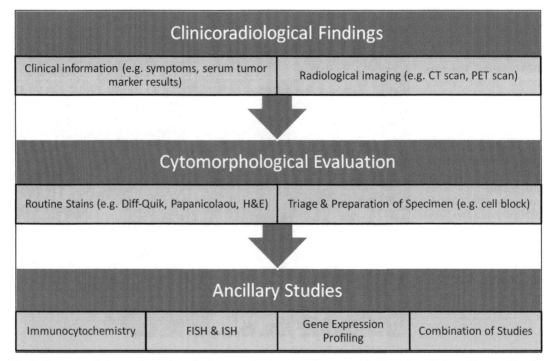

Fig. 5. Summary of diagnostic work-up for tumors of unknown primary sampled by cytopathology. The combination of clinical, radiologic, cytomorphologic, and ancillary study results in modern medicine can establish a diagnosis for most tumors without a known primary and enhance the ability to treat patients with specific site-directed therapies. H&E, hematoxylin and eosin; ISH, in-situ hybridization.

genetic abnormalities are associated with different tumors and targeted therapies, however, next-generation sequencing may introduce a new shift in the field whereby actionable

biomarkers are simply looked for without as much concern for labeling a tumor with a particular site of origin.

FUTURE TRENDS

Tumors of unknown primary represent a minority of cytologic cases due to the success of ICC, FISH, and molecular studies in addition to improved imaging and diagnostic evaluation in medicine (see **Fig. 5**). Ancillary studies have an important role in these patients not only as a diagnostic tool to determine an origin for a tumor of unknown origin but also to provide crucial prognostic and predictive information. Of these studies, ICC is the most widely used and plays a critical role in establishing accurate diagnoses and in providing important information to treating clinicians. Molecular studies are also emerging as a potentially helpful study in a subset of cases; however, these studies tend to be more costly and require more time and expertise. Moving forward, the need for determining an exact origin of a tumor may not be as critical as simply screening for potential mutations that are amenable to targeted therapies. Furthermore, as more antibodies and molecular studies are developed and applied to cytologic material, the challenges will include development of optimized and standardized

---

Key Points

PRACTICAL APPROACH TO
PATHOLOGIC EVALUATION OF TUMORS
OF UNKNOWN PRIMARY

- Obtain good clinical history and radiologic imaging findings.

- Evaluate cytomorphology to obtain preliminary differential diagnosis.

- Obtain sufficient material for ancillary studies and triage appropriately.

- Order unstained slides for potential ancillary studies upfront to avoid tissue loss.

- Use a tiered approach to ancillary studies:

  ○ ICC to determine cell type, then site-specific markers and CK7/20 profile

  ○ Molecular studies for theranostic purposes, based on ICC subtyping

- If clinical-radiologic findings and ICC are inconclusive as to the primary site of origin, consider molecular genetic profiling assays.

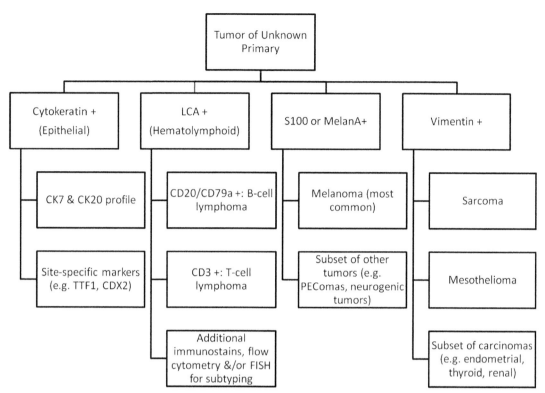

Fig. 6. Diagnostic approach using ICC to determine cell type and tumor origin.

protocols, optimization of cells available for these studies, validation of new platforms available for these studies (eg, multiplex staining), and new digital applications to enhance interpretation of the results (eg, image analysis). In addition, the development and validation of reliable immunostains to determine the mutational status of a tumor to decrease the need for more costly and time-consuming molecular studies will be a focus as well. With the application of these ancillary studies to small tissue samples, like cytology specimens, the best diagnosis can be achieved for patients with minimal tissue and, hopefully, patient care will be improved by minimizing tumors of uncertain origin and maximizing the ability to offer site-specific therapies.

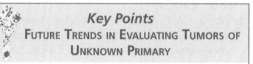

Key Points
FUTURE TRENDS IN EVALUATING TUMORS OF UNKNOWN PRIMARY

- Newer antibodies to limit the need for more costly, time-consuming molecular studies

- Optimization of protocols for different tumor types

- Optimization of processing to maximize cells available

- Improved methods for ICC with dual or multiplex staining to preserve tissue

- New platforms for interpretation of results (eg, image analysis)

- Next-generation sequencing for evaluation of biomarkers of theranostic significance

REFERENCES

1. Greco FA. Cancer of unknown primary site: evolving understanding and management of patients. Clin Adv Hematol Oncol 2012;10:518–24.
2. Tan DS, Montoya J, Ng QS, et al. Molecular profiling for druggable genetic abnormalities in carcinoma of unknown primary. J Clin Oncol 2013;31:e237–9.
3. Varadhachary GR. Carcinoma of unknown primary: focused evaluation. J Natl Compr Canc Netw 2011; 9:1406–12.
4. Varadhachary GR. New strategies for carcinoma of unknown primary: the role of tissue of origin molecular profiling. Clin Cancer Res 2013;19(15):4027–33.
5. Shaw PH, Adams R, Jordan C, et al. A clinical review of the investigation and management of carcinoma of unknown primary in a single cancer network. Clin Oncol (R Coll Radiol) 2007;19:87–95.

6. Dolled-Filhart MP, Rimm DL. Gene expression array analysis to determine tissue of origin of carcinoma of unknown primary: cutting edge or already obsolete? Cancer Cytopathol 2013;121:129–35.

7. Kamposioras K, Pentheroudakis G, Pectasides D, et al. Malignant melanoma of unknown primary site. To make the long story short. A systematic review of the literature. Crit Rev Oncol Hematol 2011;78:112–26.

8. Paholpak P, Sirichativapee W, Wisanuyotin T, et al. Prevalence of known and unknown primary tumor sites in spinal metastasis patients. Open Orthop J 2012;6:440–4.

9. Pentheroudakis G, Greco FA, Pavlidis N. Molecular assignment of tissue of origin in cancer of unknown primary may not predict response to therapy or outcome: a systematic literature review. Cancer Treat Rev 2009;35:221–7.

10. Greco FA, Spigel DR, Yardley DA, et al. Molecular profiling in unknown primary cancer: accuracy of tissue of origin prediction. Oncologist 2010;15(5):500–6.

11. Monaco SE. Cytopathology of lung cancer: moving from morphology to molecular. Diagn Histopathol 2012;18:313–20.

12. Ocque R, Tochigi N, Ohori NP, et al. Usefulness of immunohistochemical and histochemical studies in the classification of lung adenocarcinoma and squamous cell carcinoma in cytologic specimens. Am J Clin Pathol 2011;136:81–7.

13. Sigel CS, Moreira AL, Travis WD, et al. Subtyping of non-small cell lung carcinoma: a comparison of small biopsy and cytology specimens. J Thorac Oncol 2011;6:1849–56.

14. Nicholson AG, Gonzalez D, Shah P, et al. Refining the diagnosis and EGFR status of non-small cell lung carcinoma in biopsy and cytologic material, using a panel of mucin staining, TTF-1, cytokeratin 5/6, and P63, and EGFR mutation analysis. J Thorac Oncol 2010;5:436–41.

15. Rekhtman N, Brandt SM, Sigel CS, et al. Suitability of thoracic cytology for new therapeutic paradigms in non-small cell lung carcinoma: high accuracy of tumor subtyping and feasibility of EGFR and KRAS molecular testing. J Thorac Oncol 2011;6:451–8.

16. Khayyata S, Yun S, Pasha T, et al. Value of P63 and CK5/6 in distinguishing squamous cell carcinoma from adenocarcinoma in lung fine-needle aspiration specimens. Diagn Cytopathol 2009;37:178–83.

17. Mukhopadhyay S, Katzenstein AL. Subclassification of non-small cell lung carcinomas lacking morphologic differentiation on biopsy specimens: utility of an immunohistochemical panel containing TTF-1, napsin A, p63, and CK5/6. Am J Surg Pathol 2011;35:15–25.

18. Sack MJ, Roberts SA. Cytokeratins 20 and 7 in the differential diagnosis of metastatic carcinomas in cytologic specimens. Cytopathology 1997;16:132–6.

19. Ascoli V, Taccogna S, Scalzo CC, et al. Utility of cytokeratin 20 in identifying the origin of metastatic carcinomas in effusions. Diagn Cytopathol 1995;12:303–8.

20. Dejmek A, Naucler P, Smedjeback A, et al. (TA02) is a useful alternative to thyroid transcription factor-1 (TTF-1) for the identification of pulmonary adenocarcinoma cells in pleural effusions. Diagn Cytopathol 2007;35:493–7.

21. Begum S, Gillison ML, Ansari-Lari MA, et al. Detection of human papillomavirus in cervical lymph nodes: a highly effective strategy for localizing site of tumor origin. Clin Cancer Res 2003;9:6469–75.

22. Zhang MQ, El-Mofty SK, Dávila RM. Detection of human papillomavirus-related squamous cell carcinoma cytologically and by in situ hybridization in fine-needle aspiration biopsies of cervical metastasis: a tool for identifying the site of an occult head and neck primary. Cancer 2008;114:118–23.

23. Dabbs DJ, Wang X. Immunocytochemistry on cytologic specimens of limited quantity. Diagn Cytopathol 1998;18:166–9.

24. Fowler LJ, Lachar WA. Application of immunohistochemistry to cytology. Arch Pathol Lab Med 2008;132:373–83.

25. Gong Y, Symmans WF, Krishnamurthy S, et al. Optimal fixation conditions for immunocytochemical analysis of estrogen receptor in cytologic specimens of breast carcinoma. Cancer 2004;102:34–40.

26. Monaco SE, Shuai Y, Bansal M, et al. The diagnostic utility of p16 FISH and GLUT-1 immunohistochemical analysis in mesothelial proliferations. Am J Clin Pathol 2011;135:619–27.

27. Varadhachary GR, Talantov D, Raber MN, et al. Molecular profiling of carcinoma of unknown primary and correlation with clinical evaluation. J Clin Oncol 2008;26:4442–8.

28. Stancel GA, Coffey D, Alvarez K, et al. Identification of tissue of origin in body fluid specimens using a gene expression microarray assay. Cancer Cytopathol 2012;120:62–70.

29. Varadhachary GR, Spector Y, Abbruzzese JL, et al. Prospective gene signature study using microRNA to identify the tissue of origin in patients with carcinoma of unknown primary. Clin Cancer Res 2011;17:4063–70.

30. Pillai R, Deeter R, Rigl CT, et al. Validation and reproducibility of a microarray-based gene expression test for tumor identification in formalin-fixed, paraffin-embedded specimens. J Mol Diagn 2011;13:48–56.

31. Hainsworth JD, Rubin MS, Spigel DR, et al. Molecular gene expression profiling to predict the tissue of origin and direct site-specific therapy in patients with carcinoma of unknown primary site: a

Prospective Trial of the Sarah Cannon Research Institute. J Clin Oncol 2013;31:217–23.

32. Ma XJ, Patel R, Wang X, et al. Molecular classification of human cancers using a 92-gene real-time quantitative polymerase chain reaction assay. Arch Pathol Lab Med 2006;130:465–73.

33. Kerr SE, Schnabel CA, Sullivan PS, et al. Multisite validation study to determine performance characteristics of a 92-gene molecular cancer classifier. Clin Cancer Res 2012;18:3952–60.

34. Pentheroudakis G, Pavlidis N, Fountzilas G, et al. Novel microRNA-based assay demonstrates 92% agreement with diagnosis based on clinicopathologic and management data in a cohort of patients with carcinoma of unknown primary. Mol Cancer 2013;12:57.

35. Nystrom SJ, Hornberger JC, Varadhachary GR, et al. Clinical utility of gene-expression profiling for tumor-site origin in patients with metastatic or poorly differentiated cancer: impact on diagnosis, treatment, and survival. Oncotarget 2012;3:620–8.

36. Dacic S, Kothmaier H, Land S, et al. Prognostic significance of p16/cdkn2a loss in pleural malignant mesotheliomas. Virchows Arch 2008;453:627–35.

37. Sethi S, Geng L, Shidham VB, et al. Dual color multiplex TTF-1 + Napsin A and p63 + CK5 immunostaining for subcategorizing of poorly differentiated pulmonary non-small carcinomas into adenocarcinoma and squamous cell carcinoma in fine needle aspiration specimens. Cytojournal 2012;9:10.

Index

Note: Page numbers of article titles are in **boldface** type.

Surgical Pathology 7 (2014) 131–134
http://dx.doi.org/10.1016/S1875-9181(13)00143-8
1875-9181/14/$ – see front matter © 2014 Elsevier Inc. All rights reserved.

Printed and bound by CPI Group (UK) Ltd, Croydon, CR0 4YY

03/10/2024

01040309-0010